018273

KT-387-535

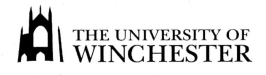

THE UNIVERSITY OF
WINCHESTER

**Martial Rose Library**
**Tel:  01962 827306**

WITHDRAWN FROM
THE LIBRARY
UNIVERSITY OF
WINCHESTER

To be returned on or before the day marked above, subject to recall.

KA 0364484 7

HALLIS

# CARE MANAGEMENT IN SOCIAL AND PRIMARY HEALTH CARE

This work was undertaken by the PSSRU, which receives support from the Department of Health; the views expressed in this publication are those of the authors and not necessarily those of the Department of Health.

# Care Management in Social and Primary Health Care
## The Gateshead Community Care Scheme

DAVID CHALLIS
*PSSRU, University of Manchester, UK*

JOHN CHESTERMAN
*PSSRU, University of Kent at Canterbury, UK*

ROSEMARY LUCKETT
*Social Services Department, Gateshead Council, UK*

KAREN STEWART
*PSSRU, University of Manchester, UK*

ROSEMARY CHESSUM
*Social Services Department, Gateshead Council, UK*

**Ashgate**

UNIVERSITY OF WINCHESTER
LIBRARY

© Personal Social Services Research Unit 2002

All rights reserved. No part of this publication may be reproduced, stored in a retrieval system or transmitted in any form or by any means, electronic, mechanical, photocopying, recording or otherwise without the prior permission of the publisher.

Published by
Ashgate Publishing Limited
Gower House
Croft Road
Aldershot
Hampshire GU11 3HR
England

Ashgate Publishing Company
131 Main Street
Burlington, VT 05401-5600 USA

Ashgate website: http://www.ashgate.com

**British Library Cataloguing in Publication Data**
Care management in social and primary health care : the
    Gateshead Community Care Scheme
    1.Social service - England - Gateshead 2.Primary care
    (Medicine) - England - Gateshead
    I.Challis, David, 1948- II.University of Kent at
    Canterbury.  Personal Social Services Research Unit
    361.3'0942873

**Library of Congress Control Number:** 2002102838

ISBN 1 85742 206 6

Typeset by Nick Brawn at the PSSRU, University of Kent at Canterbury.

Printed and bound in Great Britian by
Antony Rowe Ltd, Chippenham, Wiltshire

UNIVE⋅                    ⋅ESTER

03644847    361.3/
            CHA⋅

# Contents

# List of Boxes, Figures and Tables

# Preface

There are very many people whom we should like to thank for their contribution to this work and not all can be mentioned individually. We owe a particular debt to our colleagues closely involved in implementing and managing the programme. First the social services department staff who implemented the scheme. The care managers during the evaluation phases of the scheme, Jean Braban, Pam Royce and Jan Wilkinson, provided creative and imaginative approaches to support at home. Sheila Renton provided a very effective administrative service, developing systems to manage micro budgets. Bob Woods was responsible for the managerial initiative for the establishment and implementation of the scheme from the beginning. The NHS care managers, Carol Graham and Alyson Thomson were also creative in developing packages of care spanning the health and social care divide. Dr Ian Bowns undertook medical assessments in the health and social care scheme and was a source of infectious enthusiasm. Margaret Edwards played an important role in developing rehabilitation activities in the community. It is their work that has made the scheme a success and they are in a true sense co-authors. At the PSSRU, Nick Brawn typeset the manuscript with his usual skill.

We should like to thank the Department of Health, which funds the Personal Social Services Research Unit; the then Director, Professor Bleddyn Davies, for his personal support; and the Department of the Environment, who provided the initial funding for the social care and health and social care schemes. We are grateful to the elected members of Gateshead Metropolitan Borough for their imagination and courage in backing these initiatives and to the first Director of Social Services, Graham Lythe, for his enthusiasm, support and commitment in introducing the scheme to the department and to his successors, David Stevenson, Barry Taylor and Simon Hart for their continued support.

Dr David Henley and Lesley Longstaff, then of the health authority and community trust respectively, played an important part in developing the health and social care scheme, as did many other staff of the local health and social services.

The care scheme helpers deserve our particular thanks for their contribution in providing support to frail older people. Finally, we are especially indebted to the older people and their families who helped us by participating in careful and sometimes lengthy interviews about the difficulties they experienced in managing to cope at home in the face of extreme disability and frailty.

*David Challis, Professor of Community Care Research,*
*Director of PSSRU, University of Manchester*

*John Chesterman, Research Fellow,*
*PSSRU, University of Kent at Canterbury*

*Rosemary Luckett, formerly Team Leader,*
*Gateshead Community Care Scheme,*
*now Head of Services for Older People, Gateshead Council*

*Karen Stewart, Research Fellow,*
*PSSRU, University of Manchester*

*Rosemary Chessum, formerly Research Officer,*
*Gateshead Community Care Scheme,*
*now Area Child Protection Committee Officer, Gateshead Council*

# 1 Care Management, Coordinated and Integrated Care

There has been a longstanding concern to provide integrated and coordinated care for vulnerable older people. This is evident in the long-term care policies of many countries (Kraan et al., 1991; Challis et al., 1994; Campbell and Ikegami, 1999). In the UK, this concern can been seen to have moved from approaches which address inter agency collaboration and joint planning through the 1970s (Webb and Wistow, 1986), towards an increasing emphasis upon integration at the practice level. This is evident in such initiatives as Care in the Community (DHSS, 1981) and most obviously the White Paper *Caring for People* (Cm 849, 1989). The latter marks the point at which policy focuses both on macro and on micro level initiatives to promote these goals at the same time. In that policy document assessment and care management were framed as the cornerstone of high quality care. In the recent White Paper *Modernising Social Services* (Cm 4169, 1998) the importance of coordination, clarity of role, flexibility of services and efficiency are again stressed. Key areas for action are the promotion of independence, improving consistency and providing convenient user-centred services. These activities are set in a context of more macro level integration reflected in the development of partnerships between health and social care (Department of Health, 1998b). This is particularly evident in proposals to create care trusts and the growing leadership importance of primary care exemplified in the current emergence of primary care trusts (Cm 4818-I, 2000). Care management can thus be seen as a field level mechanism for coordinating care, which links into the more macro issues of commissioning, service development and joint working.

This book examines intensive care management for frail older people, designed to provide a realistic community-based approach to long-term care for vulnerable people.

*1*

### Current issues in care management

The contribution of care management to the long-term care of older people spans the policy agenda of the 1990s and that of the new millennium (Warburton and McCracken, 1999). However, following its introduction in mainstream social care in the UK, there appear to be a number of concerns regarding certain aspects of the approach that have been relatively poorly developed. In a review of care management implementation, as part of an evaluation of the impact of *Caring for People*, five key areas for development were identified (Challis, 1999). These were assessment; definition of care management; differentiation of care management; service development; and integrating health and social care. Each is discussed briefly below.

#### Assessment

There appears to be wide variability in assessment systems both in terms of content (what information is sought about needs and how it is recorded) and also in form (the personnel and processes involved in conducting the assessment). This remains the case even where critical decisions are being made such as whether or not a person requires residential or nursing home care. Hence, the degree of variability in assessment approaches appears to be far greater than could be attributed to the variability of the needs and circumstances of those being assessed (Stewart et al., 1999).

#### Definition of care management

There appears to be little evidence of a shared and agreed definition of care management used by agencies. In the absence of such a definition, care management may be coming to have no more meaning than the process by which people are processed through a care agency. The definition of care management provided in the official guidance on assessment and care management described care management as 'the process of tailoring services to individual needs. Assessment is an integral part of care management' (SSI/SWSG, 1991a, p. 11). Such a definition is broad and permits a wide variety of interpretations. It is in contrast to the sorts of definition which relate care management more specifically to long-term care (Applebaum and Austin, 1990; Challis, 1994a; Challis et al., 1995). As a consequence, care management in the UK more frequently represents a description of the broad variety of processes by which people are assessed and gain access to services and less a specific form of activity — coordinating care for highly vulnerable individuals. Accordingly, it may be helpful to define care management in terms of six characteristics, which distinguish it from other community-based care activities. These are the specific functions of care management; the goals it aims to achieve; the core tasks of the activity itself; the attributes of the target population; specific differentiating features; and the multi-level focus of the activity, both at practice level and system level (Challis et al., 1995).

## Differentiation of care management

In the UK in many local authorities care management is perceived as a process provided to all service users, irrespective of the intensity, severity or complexity of their needs. This is in contrast to much of the substantive research evidence on care management, which has targeted the most vulnerable older people and has been designed to shift the balance of care towards community-based support from a reliance on nursing and residential care, thereby enhancing user choice. The need to differentiate between, at the very least, care management approaches for very vulnerable people and the assessment and allocation of services to less vulnerable people has been a consistent theme in reports of the Social Services Inspectorate, following implementation of the community care reforms in 1993 (Department of Health, 1994; SSI, 1997).

Indeed, in the annual report of the Social Services Inspectorate in 1997 difficulties experienced by local authorities in coping with the volume of work were in part ascribed to a failure to differentiate between levels of intervention. It rightly concluded that no single model of care management will suit all levels of need or service user groups and identified three distinct types of care management activity, each of which was necessary for an integrated and comprehensive approach. In general terms these three approaches could be identified as screening — to provide information and advice; coordination — organising the care of a relatively large number of cases requiring relatively straightforward services; and intensive care management — where a designated care manager plans and coordinates care, undertaking a supportive role for a much smaller number of users with complex and frequently changing needs.

## Service development

The main focus of care management activity appears to have been at the level of the individual service user. Although this is an entirely right and proper focus of activity, the associated activity of service development, designed to produce more user centred services, has been much less evident. Service development may be initiated either through the micro purchasing activities of care management teams, or indirectly through feedback to those with responsibility for commissioning services from providers. Reasons why this area of activity may have been neglected include the lack of devolved budgets (Audit Commission, 1997; Challis et al., 2001).

*Integrating health and social care*

Integrating health and social care is a key theme of recent policy initiatives (Department of Health, 1997, 1998b; Cm 4169, 1998; Cm 4818-I, 2000). There is a lack of evidence of the appropriate influence of health care professionals in the assessment of older people (Challis, 1999) and even more so, a lack of evidence of the inputs from secondary health care services such as geriatric medicine and old age psychiatry. Care management systems working on a single agency basis and lacking access to appropriate expertise in assessment are unlikely to be fully effective, particularly in the care of individuals with complex problems. Integration of health and social care on the basis of differentiated care management, perhaps linking intensive care management and secondary health care, offers possibilities in the world of new care trusts (Challis et al., 1998a).

## The wider care management context

These issues are by no means confined to the UK, but in various ways are the concerns of care management and integrated care in many countries (Applebaum and Austin, 1990; Ozanne, 1990; Davies, 1992; Challis et al., 1995; Rothman and Sager, 1998). Assessment has been central to the matching of needs and resources for frail older people in many countries and the history of variation in the size and content of assessment tools would receive a ready response in many other jurisdictions. The relationship of health expertise, and particularly health care expertise, to the assessment process is also a subject of debate (Challis et al., 1998a). For example, in Australia, a concern for more appropriate targeting of cases in nursing homes is reflected in a precise focus upon the improvement of assessment processes at the point of entry to long-term care. The Aged Care Reforms of the 1980s made Aged Care Assessment Teams, which are frequently full multidisciplinary groupings, responsible for pre-placement assessment (Department of Community Services, 1986). This provided for greater consistency in the personnel undertaking assessment and, in addition, specific goals and guidelines were provided to shape the work of assessment teams (Brown and McCallum, 1991). These would be entirely within the spirit of UK current policy and were:
- To focus upon the needs and wishes of the assessed persons and their carers.
- To be able to refer to a range of services if institutional care is not deemed appropriate.
- To ensure that service users are involved in the development and management of assessment services.
- To ensure equity of access.

In terms of the integration agenda, the Australian reforms again suggest ways in which health and social care may link more effectively by providing examples of care management linked to assessment teams and based within the auspices of a health care service (Challis et al., 1995, 1998a). Finally, with regard to the issue of differentiation, there are concerns in other countries where the term care management has been employed to describe coordination of single agency activities, rather than the more circumscribed definition of long-term care case management employed by Applebaum and Austin (1990) in the USA. Thus, the nature of care management needs greater clarification (Rothman and Sager, 1998).

## Care management and the Gateshead study

The Gateshead study assumes importance through being one of the studies of care management for highly vulnerable people which were influential in shaping certain aspects of the UK community care reforms. It was explicitly cited as an exemplar of care management in the White Paper *Caring for People* (Cm 849, 1989). As such it was one of a family of demonstration studies of intensive care management targeted upon vulnerable older people, whose needs ranged from the equivalent of those living in residential care settings through nursing home and hospital residents. These studies were undertaken both as single agency approaches to intensive care management (Challis and Davies, 1986; Challis et al., 1990a) and also as joint health and social care interventions in primary health care (Challis et al., 1990a), linked to geriatric medicine (Challis et al., 1995) and old age psychiatry (Challis et al., 1997). These were designed to provide an effective and realistic alternative to institutional care for vulnerable older people, increasing the range of choice available, and are summarised in Challis (1999).

The model of care management that was developed in these initiatives was designed to ensure that improved performance of the core tasks of care management could contribute towards more effective and efficient long-term care for highly vulnerable people. The devolution of control of resources to individual care managers, within an overall cost framework, was arranged to permit more flexible response to need and the integration of fragmented services into a coherently planned pattern of care. Care managers specialised in work with highly vulnerable older people and had defined caseload limits.

There were two distinct developments within the experimental phase of the Gateshead scheme. The first was the social care scheme, a social services department initiative designed to prevent unnecessary admissions to institutional care. As such it sought to test the validity of the Kent community care project (Challis and Davies, 1986) within an urban setting. Due to the operational success of the social care scheme, additional resources were provided some four years later by central government and the health authority for a pilot health and social care scheme. This built upon the existing social care scheme, by providing a multidisciplinary care management team, including rehabilitation inputs, covering the patients of one large group practice.

In reviewing models of long-term care in the US, Kane (1999) identifies seven features that are characteristic of effective systems. Interestingly, six of these characteristics were key elements in the Gateshead programme. These were:

- A programme shaped by clearly articulated goals and values, such as independence and choice.
- A single point of access for determining eligibility, assessment and care management.
- A continuum of services and the capacity to make flexible, innovative and unorthodox care arrangements.
- Ready availability of personal care services.
- Flexibility of providers of care, including the capacity for family members to be paid providers.
- A focus not only upon safety and basic care needs, but also upon broader care goals.

### The Gateshead study and current policy developments

The Gateshead study is particularly valuable in the light of current policy for a number of reasons. First, it was cited as an exemplar of intensive care management, providing a realistic community alternative for vulnerable people, and thereby contributing to the policy goal of shifting the balance of care and increasing the range of choice (Cm 849, 1989, para. 3.3.3). In subsequent years the development of care management has provided few examples of an intensive approach to home support (Challis et al., 2001) and therefore, as policy makers and practitioners seek to develop such services the relevance of this study is increasingly evident. Second, it was one of the first approaches to care management that developed close links with primary health care. These linkages were more than an approach to case-finding and effective liaison, as has often been the case, but were more the kinds of developments that might be associated with primary care trusts today. The Gateshead initiative sought to engage medical assessment at home with joint nursing and social work care management and rehabilitative approaches in the community. Third, unlike many innovations, the scheme has in various forms been maintained over a long period of time as part of a social services organisation and continues to provide support to vulnerable older people who are more dependent than the average person entering residential and nursing home care. Its influence cannot therefore be seen as that of a short-term project. Finally, and as a consequence of the earlier three points, it provides a particularly relevant example of a number of the key concerns facing care management in the UK at the present time.

**Structure of the book**

Following this brief introductory chapter, Chapter 2 describes the service context and the research design for both the social care and the health and social care scheme. Chapters 3 to 8 provide a detailed evaluation of the social care scheme, examining in turn: care management in social care; the role of helpers commissioned by care managers; the variety of responses made to common areas of need of older people; the outcomes of the scheme for older people; the outcomes of the scheme for carers; and the costs of care and the factors that determined variation in costs. Chapter 9 examines integrated provision and the impact of the joint primary health and social care scheme. Chapter 10 reviews the lessons from the scheme for current policy and practice developments and considers how the scheme developed before, during and after the community care reforms of the 1990s.

# 2  Service Context and Research Design

This chapter is essentially in two parts. The first part describes the organisational setting in which the study was undertaken. The second part describes the research design of both the social care and health and social care schemes. In this latter section the processes of ensuring similarity between experimental and comparison groups are described, and the consequent matched groups are compared.

## Gateshead: a short history of the setting

The Metropolitan district of Gateshead, in the north-east of England, was created in the local government reorganisation of 1974 from the amalgamation of the old borough of Gateshead with some areas previously part of County Durham. At that time it had a total population of 211,333. In 1981, when the original scheme began, central Gateshead had a population of 74,644 and was the fourth largest town in County Durham. The area runs along the south bank of the river Tyne, containing areas of inner city and on the outer edge both urban and rural districts.

Gateshead as a township grew in importance during the late 11th and 12th centuries and coal mining operations and shipping developed in the 14th century. During the 15th and 16th centuries, coalfields developed in the Gateshead area and the population more than doubled. By the end of the 17th century coal mining was in decline. The economic status of the area only revived with growth in iron making and glass manufacturing and technical progress in mining. Continuing industrial expansion led to increased population with the associated social problems of poor housing and sanitation. Further growth came with the development of the railway industry, so that the population of the town increased by one third between 1820 and 1840.

Industrial decline was however evident before the First World War and this pattern continued subsequently. During the First World War much housing in central Gateshead became unfit for habitation, and in the 1920s and 1930s there was substantial growth in public sector housing. Private sector developments also took place at the same time. In 1936 a national housing survey indicated Gateshead to be one of the more deprived county boroughs in England, with 15.8 per cent of its population living in overcrowded conditions. During the inter-war years Gateshead suffered severely and in 1934 J.B. Priestley described the town as nothing better than a huge dingy dormitory. In 1936 substantial investment through the recommendations of the Commissioner for Special Areas led to the creation of the Team Valley Industrial Estate. More recently, during the early 1980s, derelict land was converted into one of Britain's largest out-of town shopping complexes, the Metro Centre. In 1990 a large tract of derelict industrial land in the Team Valley district was chosen for the setting for the 1990 National Garden Festival (Woodhouse, 1992).

### Level of service provision in the area

At the time when the scheme began, the social services department was organised into six districts covering the whole of the metropolitan borough. The internal organisation of each district varied, with social work teams deployed both on a specialist/client group basis and on a generic basis. The administrative structure of the department was along functional lines, with assistant directors responsible for fieldwork, residential care, community services and administration. As an innovation, the scheme was made organisationally responsible to the Assistant Director, Community Services, within the department.

At the commencement of the scheme there were fourteen residential care homes run by the local authority distributed throughout the borough, with an average of 40 beds each. There were also 41 residents funded by the local authority in voluntary homes, private residential homes and in facilities run by adjacent local authorities. By the late 1980s Gateshead's growth in social services expenditure per capita was above average for metropolitan boroughs, although the proportion spent upon older people aged 75 and over was below average. The number of people receiving home help was below the average, as was the number of residents aged 75 and over in residential care homes. In the borough as a whole the number of places in residential care homes was below the average of all metropolitan boroughs. Conversely, the level of home help hours received per capita was higher than the average (Department of Health, 1988).

Although close to large teaching hospitals, most of the people in the borough received their health care from hospitals within the Gateshead health district, which was nearly coterminous with the local authority. Only on the westerly margins were patients likely to enter other catchment areas for hospital care, although psychiatric inpatient care was provided in a large hospital about twenty miles away. Health care provision relied upon one major district general hospital with some services coming from two outlying hospitals. These two accounted for 46 per cent of all admissions aged 65 and over when the scheme commenced. At that time these hospitals specialised in general medicine, surgery and geriatrics. Over the period one of the hospitals became more of a long-stay facility, while the other continued to provide the same range of services. By 1987 these two hospitals accounted for only 14 per cent of all admissions aged 65 and over. At the commencement of the scheme there was also a cottage hospital unit with 30 beds and two long-stay units, with 47 and 63 beds respectively.

The Department of the Environment through the Inner Cities Partnership arrangement provided the funding for the social care scheme, including the researcher based on site. The Department of Health provided the costs of other research resources at the Personal Social Services Research Unit. The Department of the Environment through the Inner Cities Partnership also provided the funding for the additional health element of the health and social care scheme. Subsequently the scheme was funded by Gateshead social services department, and the health resources by the health authority.

## The research design

The aim of the research was to examine the kinds of care arrangements which are necessary to maintain frail older people in their own homes, to compare the impact of the scheme with standard provision on older people and their carers and to compare the costs of the scheme with standard provision. Thus, the research questions were concerned with two broad areas — care process, or how the scheme operated, and costs and effectiveness, the impact of the scheme.

The *care process* questions examine the way in which the team responded to the control of resources and greater flexibility, and the kinds of care strategies which were developed for older people with different problems.

The *costs and effectiveness* questions examine the effects of the scheme for older people and their families, compared with standard care services, and the relative costs of care.

This section describes the methods of evaluation used for the social care scheme and for the smaller health care scheme. This is followed by a description of the data collected and finally by a description of the process used to match cases receiving the scheme with those in the comparison group.

*The social care scheme*

The design of the evaluation of the social care scheme was quasi-experimental, as in the earlier study in Kent described in detail elsewhere (Challis and Davies, 1986; Davies and Challis, 1981, 1986). It is shown in Figure 2.1. In order to provide a comparison or control group for the evaluation, elderly people receiving the social care scheme were compared with a similar matched group of elderly people receiving the usual range of services from adjacent areas within Gateshead. Of the six social services districts in Gateshead, the social care scheme operated in two, both in the western part, with the three districts in the eastern part forming the comparison area. Both the experimental and comparison areas contained inner and outer city districts.

Research interviews were undertaken with older people and their carers either immediately before receipt of the scheme, or, in the case of the comparison group, when they were identified as suitable high-need comparison cases. The information collected in the interviews with older people included information about dependency and activities of daily living (Katz et al., 1963; Fillenbaum 1978), measures of social support, indicators of morale (Lawton, 1975) and depression (Snaith et al., 1971), and measures of the quality and adequacy of care provided (Challis and Davies, 1986). The schedules were based upon those employed in the Kent study, which are described in *Care Management in Community Care* (ibid.). Interviews were also undertaken with the

**Figure 2.1**
*Quasi-experimental design: social care scheme*

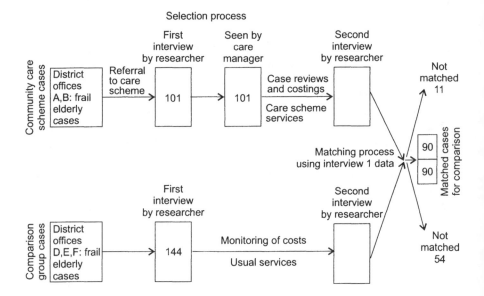

informal carers of older people, focusing on their experience of providing care and the degree of burden for them in doing so. These included a global measure of stress (Rutter et al., 1970), and indicators of burden (Challis and Davies, 1986) and of major demands upon the carer arising from the older person's needs (Grad and Sainsbury, 1968; Hoenig and Hamilton, 1969; Challis and Davies, 1986). These interviews were repeated with both groups after one year in order to identify changes in the experiences of older people and their carers as a result of receiving the different services. Case review information was completed for those older people receiving the social care scheme by the care managers at regular intervals to provide a profile of service user problems, resources used and fieldworker activities. For both groups the costs of services used were monitored over a one-year period. Following the selection of suitable cases in the experimental and comparison areas, individuals were subsequently matched on a number of factors likely to be associated with the outcome of care at home in order to provide two comparable groups of older people, similar except for the types of care they received.

### The health and social care scheme

Resources for this scheme, operating in one group practice in the western part of the borough, did not permit an experimental evaluation. However, it was possible to monitor the scheme closely by using assessment, case review and costing information completed by the case managers. This made it possible to compare the destinational outcomes and costs of older people receiving this health and social care scheme with a subset of the cases receiving existing services who had been previously identified as comparison cases in the main social care scheme. The comparative monitoring process used in the health and social care scheme is shown in Figure 2.2.

### The matching process — the social care scheme

This section describes how the social care and comparison groups were matched. The Borough of Gateshead was effectively divided into two parts for the purposes of the study, the western half being eligible for the experimental service and the eastern half providing a comparison population.

Great care was taken to identify cases in similar need in the comparison areas to those being accepted by the scheme in the experimental area. The research worker made every attempt to identify sources of referral and cases of a similar kind, nature and type of difficulty to those referred to the experimental group. Thus every effort was made to eliminate differences between the two groups of older people prior to the research interview. As a result there were 245 suitable cases included in the initial analysis. This included a greater number of comparison than experimental cases to allow for the exclusion of

**Figure 2.2**

*Comparative monitoring process: health and social care scheme*

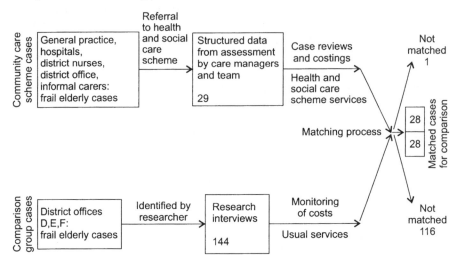

some comparison cases in creating two groups as similar as possible. Of these cases, 101 were experimental cases and 144 were comparison cases. These were examined on a wide range of different descriptive variables and initial assessments of need shown in Box 2.1.

Comparisons were made by analysis of variance and chi-square tests where appropriate, and the significant results are shown in Table 2.1. It can be seen that there are differences between the two groups that are significant at the 5 per cent level on 23 of the 61 variables. On all those indicators save one the experimental group appeared to be more dependent than the comparison group. On measures of disability, problems with activities of daily living and health the experimental group experienced greater difficulty. This was, of course, not surprising given the greater difficulty of identifying comparison group cases in the high dependency category. The only measure indicating greater need in the comparison group was a count of the number of extra services required. The explanation for this appeared to be that the comparison group cases, being less disabled, were able to make use of a wider range of services such as day care or lunch clubs which were less appropriate for the experimental group.

In order to achieve greater similarity between the two populations, so as to ensure that at the onset of the study there was as little variation as possible between the two groups, a process of matching was undertaken. By carefully matching individual cases it was hoped to eliminate much of the variance between the groups.

## Box 2.1
*Variables used in comparing experimental and control groups before and after matching*

### 1. Initial matching criteria
Age
Gender
Dependency (interval measure of
    need)
Presence of informal carer
Living group
Attitude to help

### 2. Social support
Loneliness
Social contacts
Social Resources Rating (OARS)[a]

### 3. Activities of daily living
*Need for help with:*
    getting into bed
    getting up
    washing
    dressing
    feeding
    toileting
    getting about in home
    getting outside home
    getting in and out of chair
    avoiding self neglect
    managing medication
    bathing or showering
    cutting toenails
    with light housework
    making hot drink/snack
    making a hot meal
    managing fire/heating system
    managing heavy housework
    doing shopping
    managing laundry
    managing soiled linen
    managing garden
Activities of Daily Living rating
    (OARS)[a]
Activities of Daily Living Index (Katz
    et al.)[b]

### 4. Physical and mental health
Self rated health
Eyesight problems
Hearing problems
Breathlessness
Giddiness
Risk of falling
Incontinence of urine
Incontinence of faeces
Depression Index
Depression rating
Anxiety rating
Memory score
Confusional state rating
Mental Health Resources rating
    (OARS)[a]
Physical Health Resources rating
    (OARS)[a]
Memory and behaviour score

### 5. Outcome measures
Need for additional help rising and re-
    tiring
Need for additional help with personal
    care during the day
Need for additional help with daily
    household activities
Need for additional help with weekly
    household activities
Felt capacity to cope
Morale score
Need for extra services

### 6. Other factors
Housing suitability
Receipt of supplementary benefits
Economic Resources rating (OARS)[a]
Recent bereavement
Whether going out weekly

a  Fillenbaum (1978)
b  Katz et al. (1963)

**Table 2.1**
*Significant differences between the groups and mean values before matching*

| Variable | Experimental | | Comparison |
|---|---|---|---|
| *Needs help with:* | | | |
| getting up | 2.38 | * | 2.18 |
| washing | 2.50 | ** | 2.24 |
| dressing | 2.62 | *** | 2.29 |
| toileting | 2.68 | ** | 2.39 |
| getting around outside | 3.51 | ** | 3.29 |
| bathing | 3.54 | *** | 3.11 |
| toenails | 3.67 | *** | 3.28 |
| daily housework | 3.20 | *** | 2.87 |
| making hot drink/snack | 3.01 | * | 2.82 |
| making hot meal | 3.58 | * | 3.40 |
| managing fire/heating appliance | 2.81 | ** | 2.48 |
| heavy housework | 3.97 | *** | 3.78 |
| shopping | 3.84 | *** | 3.65 |
| laundry | 3.74 | *** | 3.44 |
| soiled linen | 2.70 | ** | 2.19 |
| Risk of falling | 1.48 | * | 1.28 |
| Incontinence of urine | 0.81 | * | 0.62 |
| Incontinence of faeces | 0.67 | *** | 0.38 |
| Need for extra services | 8.67 | *** | 10.03 |
| Activities of daily living (OARS)[a] | 4.88 | *** | 4.51 |
| Need for help rising and retiring | 5.93 | *** | 4.99 |
| Need for help with daily housework | 4.58 | *** | 3.17 |
| Number of times going out during week | 1.08 | *** | 2.31 |

* $p < 0.05$; ** $p < 0.01$; *** $p < 0.001$
a Fillenbaum (1978)

The method of matching cases was developed from the initial study of the community care scheme in Kent (Challis and Davies, 1985, 1986). The objective was to match the cases by a combination of different variables, which were likely to be predictors of outcome in the care of older people. The seven variables used were the degree of dependency of the older person, household structure (living group), the degree of mental impairment suffered by the older person, the presence or absence of an informal carer, the older person's age, gender and apparent attitude to receipt of help. They are listed in Box 2.2. Each is examined in more detail below.

The living group variable was initially based upon a differentiation between those older people living alone and those living with others. The presence of an informal carer was assessed by the interviewer who identified whether there was a carer or not. Dependency was assessed using the method of Isaacs and Neville (1976) which was dependent upon the degree to which the older person could be left to manage alone without requiring further help. This

**Box 2.2**
*Variables used in the matching process*

**Age**
Below 75
75 to 84
85 plus

**Gender**
Male
Female

**Dependency**
Long Interval Need
Short Interval Need
Critical Interval Need

**Confusional State**
None/mild
Moderate/severe

**Informal carer**
Present
Absent

**Living group**
Alone
With others (spouse; other
  same age; other younger)

**Attitude to help**
Rejecting – hostile
Rejecting/unwilling – needs
  persuasion
Accepting
Dependent – demanding
Dependent – passive

provided three categories of need: critical interval need, where help was required at frequent intervals during the day; short interval need, where help was required on two or three occasions during the day, such as at meal times; and long interval need, where help was required once a day or less frequently. Age was divided into three categories. Those below 75, those between 75 and 84, and those aged 85 and over. Mental impairment was assessed by an interviewer rating of the presence of confusional state on a four-point scale that consisted of none, mild, moderate, or severe. This four-point scale was collapsed into two: those with none, or with evidence of mild confusion, were placed in the first group; and those with moderate and severe confusion in the second. Attitude to help was a five-point rating on the apparent attitude of the older person to receipt of help. It consisted of those who were independent and rejecting of help, those who were independent and required persuasion, those who were currently normally accepting of help, and those whose attitude was dependent and who were very demanding, and finally those who appeared dependent but passive.

There were two stages in the matching process, each broken into several steps. For the first stage, on the basis of these seven variables, cases were allocated by computer analysis into a number of different groups, which consisted of varying numbers of experimental and comparison group cases. These clusters or groups of cases were then individually examined by the research interviewer who identified the most appropriate individuals to match with one another within each small cluster. In this way, it was possible to undertake a more sensitive process of matching than would otherwise have been the case, simply relying upon the computer combinations. With this secondary 'clinical' process, choices could be made between possible pairs enabling a wide range of other variables to be considered. For example, the living group variable was made more subtle in this process of clinical matching and took account of those living alone, those living with a spouse, and those living with other relatives and whether those relatives were of a similar age or younger. Several other factors were also taken into account at this stage. For example, the characteristics of carers were made as similar as possible by differentiating between the carer who was physically active and providing support and someone who was also physically frail and less able to provide help. Family relationships were also taken into account by matching individuals with fairly substantial caring family networks. This made it possible to differentiate between those older people with a sole carer, from those whose carer was part of a wider network of care. It was also possible to take into account the presence of particular conditions, such as arthritis or sensory impairment, or of subtle variations within categories of physical dependency. Other individual factors were also considered, such as pairing individuals who were similar with regard to the presence of anxiety and the propensity to seek support. Again, different causal factors of apparently similar levels of dependency, some predominantly physical, others related to mental health, were taken into account. As a result of this process, it was possible to identify 60 pairs of cases who were perfectly matched by the computer criteria and subsequently matched on a clinical basis.

The second step involved the simplification of the attitude to help variable. This involved discriminating between those who were independent and rejecting, those who were relatively dependent and those who were relatively accepting of help. As a result of this process, another fourteen matched pairs were identified. Finally this indicator, being considered the least reliable, was relaxed altogether. This yielded five further pairs. Alternatives were then made to the age categories so that those under 75 were differentiated from those aged 75 and over. A further three pairs were identified in this process.

It should be noted that this was initially a computerised stepwise process involving the stages described and then subsequently individual matching was applied to the computer group selection process, choosing individuals within the selected groups but rejecting many possible pairs identified by the computer as unsuitable for other reasons. Of the 91 possible pairs identified by this process using the computer, only 75 were finally selected. Fifty-three of these 75 cases were perfect matches in that they fitted by all the criteria specified, including all five categories on the attitude to help variable.

Finally, the remaining cases were individually scrutinised using the variables already known plus a range of other health, dependency and social support variables in order to identify further possible matches. At this point, the attitude to help variable had been relaxed completely although other individual factors were taken into account. The focus was upon similarity of care problems generated by the older person's dependency. For example, the assessor in matching cases at this stage took particular care to examine cases where apparently similar dependency levels were complicated by quite different causal factors such as depressed mood on the one hand and physical illness on the other.

Similarly, some cases appeared marginal to the category in which they were placed. Carefully sifting this information identified another fifteen matched pairs. Table 2.2 lists the number of pairs in which there were differences on a particular matching variable. Thus, from 101 older people who received the social care scheme and 144 who received the usual range of services it was possible to identify 90 matched pairs of individuals for comparative purposes.

These matched cases were tested like the whole group for their similarity on a range of important descriptive and initial measures of outcome variables. The results are shown in Table 2.3. It can be seen that a number of the original differences between the groups were either eliminated or reduced. In particular, differences in the Activities of Daily Living Index, dependency group categories, and need for help with getting up, washing, dressing, using the toilet, preparing meals and snacks or hot drinks were eliminated. Symptomatic health factors such as risk of falling and urinary incontinence no longer differentiated the groups. Nevertheless, there were, as would be expected from an examination of such a number and wide range of variables, some remaining differences between the experimental and comparison groups.

Overall, the experimental group tended to be more dependent and frail than the comparison population, reflecting the difficulty of recruiting cases of a similar level of dependency to those referred to an available new service, since alternative action, such as entry to residential or hospital care is often speedily taken. It was decided that these 90 matched pairs provided an acceptable basis for comparison of the relative effectiveness of the new scheme, since

**Table 2.2**
*Cases matched by computer criteria and 'clinical' judgement*

| | |
|---|---|
| *Stage one — computer selection plus 'clinical' judgement* | |
| Matched by all criteria | 60 |
| Simplifying attitude to help indicator | 7 |
| Relaxing attitude to help criteria | 5 |
| Simplifying age criteria | 3 |
| Total | 75 |
| *Stage two — 'clinical' judgement while maximising similarity on original variables* | |
| Earlier selected cases | 75 |
| Relaxing age criterion alone | 9 |
| Relaxing gender criterion alone | 1 |
| Relaxing confusional state criterion alone | 2 |
| Relaxing dependency criterion alone | 1 |
| Modifying principal carer criterion alone | 1 |
| Relaxing age and confusional state | 1 |
| Total | 90 |

**Table 2.3**
*Significant differences between the groups and mean values after matching*

| Variable | Experimental | | Comparison |
|---|---|---|---|
| *Needs help with:* | | | |
| dressing | 2.54 | * | 2.43 |
| getting around outside | 3.57 | * | 3.37 |
| bathing | 3.58 | *** | 3.20 |
| toenails | 3.68 | * | 3.46 |
| with daily housework | 3.25 | ** | 2.97 |
| with heavy housework | 3.99 | *** | 3.82 |
| with shopping | 3.86 | *** | 3.63 |
| with laundry | 3.75 | ** | 3.51 |
| Incontinence of faeces | 0.71 | ** | 0.42 |
| Need for extra services | 8.60 | *** | 10.07 |
| Activities of daily living (OARS)[a] | 4.92 | * | 4.67 |
| Need for help rising and retiring | 6.01 | * | 5.34 |
| Need for help with daily housework | 4.65 | * | 3.43 |
| No. of times going out during week | 1.01 | ** | 2.00 |

* $p < 0.05$; ** $p < 0.01$; *** $p < 0.001$
a Fillenbaum (1978)

the effect of the remaining differences would tend to bias results against the experimental service. It is interesting to note that in the Kent Study (Challis and Davies, 1986) there were 74 matched pairs, a utilisation rate of 71 per cent. In this study 90 matched pairs were obtained, out of 245 cases, a utilisation rate of 73 per cent. The similarity is quite striking, particularly as a more sensitive approach to matching cases was employed, using seven variables instead of six, one of which was divided into three categories rather than two, and a 'clinical' process was also used.

*Comparison of the carers*

Although the individual characteristics of carers were not used as criteria in the selection of matched pairs, the groups were compared for differences in these characteristics, both before and after matching. The effect of the matching process is shown in Tables 2.4 and 2.5, after comparison of the groups for a wide range of differences. It can be seen from Table 2.4 that prior to matching, fifteen of these variables showed significant differences between the groups. Roughly twice the proportion of comparison group carers lived with the older person and they spent more time performing caring tasks. Furthermore, fewer received help from statutory services in caring for the older person. Conversely, those in the experimental group experienced more behavioural problems, had less time to spend with their spouse, suffered more anxiety and had higher degrees of strain and consequent tension within the home.

**Table 2.4**

*Significant differences between the groups regarding informal carer characteristics before matching*

| Variable | Mean value/ percentage: experimental group | Significance level of group difference | Mean value/ percentage: comparison group |
|---|---|---|---|
| Older person lives with carer | 14% | * | 29% |
| Hours/week spent by carer and family performing tasks | 30 | * | 42 |
| *Aspects of older person's behaviour causing problems* | | | |
| a. Uncooperative/personality conflicts | 1.46 | ** | 1.16 |
| b. Older person requiring nursing/ physical care | 1.72 | *** | 1.27 |
| c. Older person at risk of falling | 1.59 | * | 1.34 |
| d. Incontinence of urine | 0.79 | * | 0.52 |
| e. Incontinence of faeces | 0.63 | * | 0.39 |
| *Help received by carer and family* | | | |
| a. Help from statutory agencies — personal care | 65% | ** | 41% |
| b. Help from statutory agencies — housework/shopping | 78% | * | 61% |
| c. Help from statutory agencies — moral support | 66% | *** | 31% |
| d. Help from voluntary agencies — personal care | 1% | * | 11% |
| *Effects upon self and family* | | | |
| a. Spent less time with spouse | 2.03 | * | 1.72 |
| b. Feels worried/anxious all the time | 80% | * | 64% |
| Overall rating of strain upon helper | 2.06 | * | 1.70 |
| Overall rating of tension in home | 1.14 | * | 0.89 |
| Sample size interviewed | 71 | | 100 |
| Cases with informal carer not interviewed | 1 | | 4 |

* p <0.05; ** p <0.01; *** p <0.001
For continuous/quasi-continuous variables, significance levels were obtained using a one-way analysis of variance.
For variables with only two values, significance levels were obtained from a chi-squared test.

It can be seen from Table 2.5 that after matching there were only four significant differences between the groups, although two of these had not been present earlier, namely whether or not the older person was related to the carer and night-time disturbance. These latter two factors, one being stronger in each

**Table 2.5**
*Significant differences between the groups regarding informal carer characteristics after matching*

| Variable | Mean value/ percentage: experimental group | Significance level of group difference | Mean value/ percentage: comparison group |
|---|---|---|---|
| Whether carer unrelated to older person | 25 | * | 10 |
| *Aspects of older person's behaviour causing problems* | | | |
| a.  Noisy at night or wandering | 0.42 | * | 0.75 |
| *Help received by carer and family* | | | |
| a.  Help from statutory agencies — personal care | 67% | ** | 43% |
| b.  Help from statutory agencies — moral support | 70% | *** | 37% |
| Sample size interviewed | 64 | | 60 |
| Cases with informal carer not interviewed | 1 | | 4 |

* p <0.05; ** p <0.01; *** p <0.001

Although the matching process had been successful in making the numbers with an informal carer in each group almost the same (65 and 64), a few of these informal carers were not interviewed, making the size of each interviewed group slightly different (64 and 60).

For continuous/quasi-continuous variables, significance levels were obtained using a one-way analysis of variance.

For variables with only two values, significance levels were obtained from a chi-squared test.

group, are likely to have effects that could even out differences, possession of either attribute tending to militate against ability to be cared for at home.

### The matching process — health and social care scheme

Twenty-nine older people receiving the health and social care scheme were matched with the most frail of the 144 comparison group cases. During the period of monitoring there were in fact 33 older people who received this scheme. Four of these have been excluded from the comparison, three of them because they were specifically accepted for terminal care and were thus not comparable with comparison group cases and one case because there were insufficient data for matching. Since there were no research interviews undertaken with older people in the health and social care scheme, the data to permit matching was taken from the standardised assessment form used by the practitioners for this scheme. Using these data, cases were matched according to gender, living group (household composition), confusional state, incontinence, activities of daily living (whether or not needing help with feeding, toileting, transfer, dressing and meal preparation) and loneliness. This process provided 28 matched pairs for comparison, as shown in Figure 2.2. Following the matching, there appeared to be a close concordance between the groups and where there was a suggestion of difference it again appeared that those receiving the health and social care scheme were the more impaired. Hence, with regard to factors such as probability of entry to high cost care settings, the bias would again seem to be against this experimental group. All aspects of the health and social care scheme are examined in Chapter 9.

# 3 Care Management in the Social Care Scheme

As noted in Chapter 1, care management was identified as one of the corner-stones of community care. A considerable degree of guidance was offered from central government, both about the nature of care management and assessment (SSI/SWSG, 1991a,b) and, more generally, in a variety of circulars and advisory material, about the service context within which care management should take place. This latter included material on purchasing and contracting and community care plans. A useful and consolidated description of the implementation process can be found in Gostick et al. (1997). Nonetheless, despite guidance, there was wide room for interpretation of what different forms of care management were appropriate or necessary for which groups of people, with a consequent diversity of response in interpretation.

A number of studies have looked at post 1993 implementation of care management in the UK. The Social Services Inspectorate undertook two monitoring studies, one on assessment and the other on care management. Firstly, there was a joint SSI/NHSME study of assessment procedures in five local authority areas (Department of Health, 1993). The overarching finding from this study was that, although the new community care reforms had been successfully introduced, the assessment documentation and procedures were overly complex and time consuming. In terms of the information collected, both content and quality varied and there was a lack of reliability and validity. It was also noted that generic documentation was ill suited to identifying the needs of specific service user groups. The purpose of assessment documents was unclear — whether it was to guide assessors, demonstrate their accountability or involve the service user. Furthermore, more involvement of health care staff appeared to be needed in assessment. In terms of the content of assessment documentation the study concluded that the categorisation of needs and problems was poor and that there was no evidence of clear links between problem identification and response formulation.

Several of these observations were confirmed in more local studies which raise the importance of the relationship between assessment documents and the provision of the requisite skills and training (Caldock, 1993). It has also been noted that assessment tools tend to focus upon the functional domains and financial aspects with consequently less attention to other areas, such as mental health (Caldock, 1994; Lewis et al., 1995). Evidence from a survey of care management in Wales suggested that assessment forms were felt to be inadequate for three reasons. First, that they failed to cover all areas of need; second, many did not assess the carer's perspective; and third, the information was often not sufficient for providers to organise detailed care, and did not facilitate the construction of care plans (Parry-Jones and Caldock, 1995). A larger scale study of the content of assessment documentation confirmed these issues (Stewart et al., 1999).

The SSI care management study conducted in seven local authority areas in the following year (Department of Health, 1994) highlighted further issues of concern arising from the implementation of the community care legislation. In particular, the early focus on the creation of appropriate organisational structures, whilst understandable, had often been achieved at the expense of strategic decisions relating to the goals of care management. Of particular concern was the tendency towards rigid separation of purchaser and provider roles and the consequent effect on the development of care management practice. Whilst the latter was occurring against a backcloth of a growing specialisation in social work with specific service user groups, a discernible trend towards an administrative form of care management, characterised by a lack of continuity of staff involvement in the tasks of care management, was apparent. Linked to this was the observation that care management was becoming a process applied to all service users rather than being targeted on the more complex, volatile cases, as was the case in the studies cited in the White Paper (Cm 849, 1989). Finally, it was noted that the devolution of budgets to allow care managers to purchase care was effective when evident but that to achieve it required adequate financial monitoring systems to be in place, which were often lacking. This issue was again noted by the Audit Commission (1997), and a national study of care management (Challis et al., 1998b). A later SSI study concluded that marked variety in arrangements remained. The areas of greatest difference included screening, who does assessment whether this varies with complexity, direct access by health staff of social care resources, budget devolution, information provided to assessor/budget holder, person responsible for monitoring/review, cases reviewed and feedback to commissioning (Department of Health, 1998a).

A number of small-scale studies have indicated a marked bias in care management implementation towards a focus upon assessment and eligibility decisions to the detriment of more long-term support (Lewis, 1994; Petch et al.,

1994; Phillips, 1996). Nonetheless, Lewis et al. in their study of four authorities suggest improvements had occurred in the assessment process (Lewis et al., 1997). Another area commonly cited has been the problematic relationship between social work and care management. At times this is manifest in staff dissatisfaction with bureaucratic aspects of work associated with administration and care packaging (Lewis and Glennerster, 1996; Lewis et al., 1997), and at other times in the perceived diminution of time spent in more traditional casework activities (Hoyes et al., 1994; Pahl, 1994). As a consequence, there has been some considerable debate about the nature of social work and its relationship to care management (Parton, 1994; Payne, 1995; Sheppard, 1995). More generally, there has been uncertainty in relation to the organisational position of care management and the nature and locus of the purchaser/provider split (Hoyes et al., 1994). Lewis and Glennerster (1996) noted the need to link the process of organisational change with the precise objectives of care management if the changes were to be effective, which reflects the SSI study (Department of Health, 1994). A number of studies have identified a degree of confusion about the nature of, and the target group for, care management (Hoyes et al., 1994; Lewis and Glennerster, 1996; Petch, 1996). Although several studies and commentators have noted the importance of budgetary devolution for flexible, user and market sensitive purchasing by care managers, Lewis et al. (1995) noted the contradictory pressures to centralise budgetary control, particularly as resources became more stretched. A national study noted a high degree of variation in care management arrangements between different local authorities on a wide variety of criteria (Challis et al., 1998b).

It is clear from the very consistency of these diverse studies that there is a vagueness as to the way care management has been interpreted by different local authorities. In part this reflects the predominance of a broad definition in the guidance, which stressed activities of tailoring resources to need and the performance of a set of core tasks, such as assessment and care planning. It has been argued elsewhere that these features are necessary but not sufficient conditions for a definition of care management. A more robust definition of care management is a multi-faceted one (Challis et al., 1995). This definition is reproduced in Box 3.1 and distinguishes care management in relation to functions, goals, core tasks, target group, features differentiating it from other community-based practice, and the multi-level response of care management.

The greater need for clarity in definition was reinforced in the Sixth annual report of the Chief Inspector of Social Services, which stressed the need for a more clearly differentiated set of care management arrangements (SSI, 1997). It indicated that problems experienced by social service departments in terms of volume and flow of work could be more effectively managed by a clearer differentiation between levels of intervention. Three types or styles of care management were identified, each being appropriate for different levels of response. Together the range and breadth of responses would be necessary for an integrated and comprehensive approach to providing care. These levels were:

---

**Box 3.1**
*The key characteristics of care management*

**Functions** — coordination and linkage of care services.

**Goals** — Providing continuity and integrated care; increased opportunity for home-based care; promote client well-being; making better use of resources.

**Core tasks** — Case-finding and screening; assessment; care planning; monitoring and review; case closure.

**Characteristics of recipients** — Long-term care needs; multiple service need.

**Differentiating features** — Intensity of involvement; breadth of services spanned; lengthy duration of involvement.

**Multi-level response** — Linking practice-level activities with broader resource and agency-level activities.

---

- the administrative type, undertaken by reception and/or customer service staff, provides information and advice;
- the coordinating type that deals with a large volume of referrals needing either a single service or a range of fairly straightforward services which should be properly planned and administered; and
- the intensive type where there is a designated care manager who combines the planning and coordination with a therapeutic, supportive role for a much smaller number of users who have complex and frequently changing needs.

(SSI, 1997, para 3.4)

The main problem in the lack of effective care management arrangements was judged to arise from the failure to discriminate between the coordinating and intensive forms of care management. The Gateshead scheme fits well within this set of more differentiated arrangements. It provides a particularly clear example of a model of intensive care management, which can be considered to be a secondary level of social care response to need, rather than a primary level of care, which is the first point of service for people in need (Challis et al., 1998b). By many of the criteria which have proved problematic in the implementation of care management, the Gateshead scheme, albeit a pilot study which commenced in the 1980s, was well ahead of its time. It addressed a number of key issues, in particular, differentiated response, budgetary devolution, cost recording and monitoring, systematic assessment, a clearly specified purchasing role for care managers, and a coherent role for social work within care management.

## The model of care management in the scheme

The community care approach developed in Gateshead built upon the studies in Kent and elsewhere (Challis and Davies, 1980, 1985, 1986; Davies and

Challis, 1986; Challis, 1994b). It was designed to enable care managers to develop sensitive and appropriate alternatives to residential, nursing and long-term hospital care for frail older people. It involved the decentralisation of control of resources to individual practitioners to act as care managers with defined caseload and expenditure limits to ensure accountability, so that more flexible responses to need could be devised and the fragmented services integrated into a more coherent individual package of care. This approach to intensive care management aimed to improve the content of services through greater flexibility of response and to improve the coordination and appropriateness of care through a designated care manager. The main features of the approach are summarised in Box 3.2.

---

**Box 3.2**
*The community care approach: aims and inputs of the scheme*

**Scheme aims**

1. Improved care management.
2. Increased accountability.
3. More effective and efficient use of resources.

**Scheme characteristics**

1. Clear and continuing case responsibility.
2. Targeted caseload; fieldworker specialisation by client group.

3. Smaller caseloads.
4. Trained and experienced fieldworkers.
5. Decentralised budget, with clear expenditure limits.
6. Knowledge of unit costs of services.
7. Service packages costed.
8. Systematic records for assessment and monitoring.

---

Clear and unambiguous case responsibility exercised by designated care managers was seen as essential to avoid fragmentation of care and provide an opportunity for staff to learn from the outcome of different strategies for different kinds of problem. The caseload was defined, targeted upon the most frail older people whose needs placed them on the margin of entry to long term institutional care. The care managers had smaller caseloads, about 25-30 cases, and were recruited as being more trained/experienced than was common in work with older people, reflecting the needs and problems of these service users and the responsibility of the work. The care managers controlled a budget that could be used to purchase or develop additional services beyond those currently available, to permit a wider range of response to service users' needs. In making care decisions they were aware of the unit costs of other services, since the overall weekly level of expenditure upon a package of care for an individual was costed and limited to two-thirds of the cost of a place in a residential home. This amount reflected the approximate 'care costs' of that setting. Expenditure upon an individual case beyond this was allowed, but required line management sanction. This expenditure limit and the targeted caseload were designed to provide clear boundaries within which the potential for creative autonomy on the part of the care managers could be resolved with the need for accountability, with the expenditure acting as one trigger for management consultation. The record system served to enhance this accountability and consisted of three main elements: assessment information covering the need circumstances of older people; the use of a structured case review at least four times a year covering care manager activities, service user problems and the range of resources deployed; and weekly costings of the care packages for each older person. The records permitted summary feedback to be given about caseloads, the mix of service user problems, care manager activities and costs (Challis and Chesterman, 1986). Using this information at different levels of aggregation provided the basis for a performance management system. These organisational arrangements were designed to make effective care management possible within an accountable organisation and thereby contribute to greater efficiency in social care. Further details may be found in Challis and Davies (1986) and Davies and Challis (1986).

This approach to care management requires the care manager to undertake both direct work with the older people and their carers and indirect work in mobilising and coordinating services. As such, it is closer to clinical care management (Harris and Bergman, 1987; Kanter, 1989) than some of the more administrative approaches, which have focused principally upon effective arrangement of services.

Box 3.3 summarises the key features of the Gateshead social care scheme in relation to a set of key dimensions of care management (Challis, 1994a; Challis et al., 1995, 1998b). These indicators are: targeting; the distinction between care management and intensive care management; the location of care management; the style of care management; operational aspects of care management, such as caseload size, staff mix and continuity of care; the degree of influence over service providers; management, standards and quality assurance; and the logical coherence of care management arrangements (Challis, 1994a,b).

Davies (1992) has identified four other classificatory dimensions: direct versus indirect; administrative v. clinical; service-led v. holistic; and professional v. consumer-led. The first of these refers to the extent to which there is division in the performance of the core tasks of care management for given cases, both within and between agencies. Thus, it often reflects both the relative power of care management and the degree of continuity of care management activity. Evidence suggests that division of labour between practitioners or between agencies, an indirect model, is associated with poorer outcomes for more complex cases (Eggert et al., 1990, 1991). The administrative v. clinical dimension has been discussed earlier. Service-led care management refers to where assessment is orientated towards defining eligibility for services, rather than a more general identification of needs or problems. Clearly, whilst such models may be prevalent the new culture of community care was designed to

---

**Box 3.3**

*Key characteristics of care management in the social care scheme*

**Target group** — Older people at risk of admission to residential or nursing home care.

**Intensiveness of care management role** — Intensive care management for a high-need group.

**Location** — Social service department care managers, in specialist SSD team.

**Style of care management** — Care managers with responsibility for assessment, counselling, advice and social support, arranging, coordinating, reviewing and developing services and gap-filling.

**Operational features:**

Caseload size — small, 25-30 cases per care manager.

Staff mix — trained social workers and a community worker as care managers.

Continuity of care — long-term responsibility; undertaking all core tasks from screening to review.

**Influence over providers** — Substantial budget for purchase of external services and items; limited influence to negotiate with in-house providers.

**Management: standards and quality assurance** — Care management team manager carrying reduced caseload; own assessment, review and costs information system; supervision and review using assessment and costs information.

**Coherence of arrangements** — Integrated service model for high need group; lack of direct health care expertise in team.

---

shift attention away from this approach. The professional v. consumer-led dimension refers to the degree of consumer involvement, at its furthest pole reflected in direct payment arrangements. The Gateshead scheme, by these criteria, would be seen as a direct model of care management with a clinical orientation, a more holistic approach, although predominantly professionally-led. A brief experiment occurred in the early phase of the scheme, whereby a small amount of the care management budget was made available to social workers in one of the areas for them to act as care managers with a small number of their cases. This did not prove successful in that part-time care managers were not in a position to shift their focus of activity to a long-term care orientation and towards manoeuvring resources in new ways. The difficulties of part-time care management have also been observed elsewhere (Kendig et al., 1992).

The social care scheme commenced with the appointment of staff in late 1980 and the uptake of the first cases in early 1981. The scheme was operated as an additional resource within the social services department, and consisted of a team leader and two social workers based in their own office with secretarial support organisationally distinct from the area teams who were the first point of referral. Thus it was a secondary, specialist service concerned only with the most frail older people (Challis et al., 1998a). During the period of evaluation the team was directly responsible to an assistant director. Therefore it had fewer tiers of management then the district teams.

The team leader had a background in social work with older people, and had undertaken post-qualifying training in this field. She had had practice experience in hospital social work, including in a University department of geriatric medicine and as a specialist practitioner in an area team. Both the other two care managers were particularly interested in work with older people, one being newly qualified from social work training and the other with considerable experience of community work within the social services department. The team had its own administrator who was integral to the work of the team and the research worker was also located with the team.

**Setting up the care management service**

The initial tasks for the newly appointed care managers were to establish the legitimacy of their role and of the scheme, to ensure that they were clear about the different style of working which they were expected to develop, and to ensure that the various operational procedures necessary for effective working were developed and in place. These issues are discussed below.

*Induction and exchanging ideas from previous experience*

In order that the care managers could build upon the experience of those who had worked in the field in a similar service a week was spent in seminars and discussion sessions at the University of Kent with practitioners from Kent and North Wales who were currently engaged in providing a care management service to vulnerable older people in those areas. These discussions focused upon a whole range of practice issues, such as assessment, planning care, managing devolved budgets and solving particularly intractable care problems such as the support of older people with dementia.

*Management group*

A management group was established to ensure that different parties with an interest in the scheme were involved in decision making, problem solving and support for the service. This was convened and chaired by the assistant director responsible for the scheme. The group consisted of the assistant director, team leader, research officer, two of the district social service managers and a research manager from the University of Kent. This structure was seen as necessary to link a centrally managed innovation with senior management to keep the scheme on course, and avoid isolation and loss of the original goals while linking it into the local operational structures for effective liaison. The need for such senior management involvement and support was deemed important to retain the integrity of an innovatory service and to resolve problems arising from boundary disputes. Therefore, the scheme had a relatively short line of accountability from assistant director to team leader and had visible senior management commitment and involvement. Contact took place not only at planned meetings but also informally which was important in demonstrating senior management interest in the scheme and providing support to the staff.

## Accommodation and secretarial resources

The scheme was not able to appoint its own secretarial staff immediately until such time as the demand for such work was seen as sufficient to justify this expenditure. This meant that existing secretarial resources had to be used by the team in developing their own record and filing systems and for the sake of effective working relationships were naturally reluctant to make excessive demands on these resources. Further problems were occasioned by the need for suitable office accommodation, itself scarce, and two moves were experienced before the scheme could settle into suitable accommodation with their own administrative staff in an area closely accessible to their client catchment area after nearly eleven months. This did not contribute to the capacity of the new service to settle quickly in a stable pattern of working. The difficulties did certainly however contribute to a team spirit, a resilience and willingness to solve problems among team members.

## Role legitimacy and turf issues

Inevitably, a number of existing social services staff were ambivalent about the development of the scheme. On the one hand, the provision of extra resources to enable frail older people to remain at home was welcomed, but on the other hand, some staff saw themselves as the appropriate ones to provide this kind of service rather than the scheme. One view expressed was that such specialist social workers constituted a form of elitism, and district social work managers, probably worried about a centrally managed initiative in their areas, expressed concern about transfer of case responsibility to the care management team saying that social workers would not wish to relinquish their cases. The home help service saw none of the proposals as new, believing that domiciliary care organisers were already undertaking comprehensive assessments, and that home helps were doing all that was needed. This perception indicated a lack of appreciation that existing services, while involving the best efforts of those involved, did not cover all needs and problems. As the main budget holder for community support of older people such a new service, albeit small, was viewed by the home help service as a potential future competitor for their budget. Certainly the creation of a new service at least implicitly criticised existing services and was perceived as a threat. Nursing officers also expressed disquiet about frail older people remaining in their own homes and were specifically concerned that this would result in community nursing having a longer term involvement. Other staff were not always in agreement with the philosophy of increasing home care and housing wardens in particular perceived long-term contact between care managers and residents on estates as bypassing their role. In the face of such conflicting views, anxieties were dealt with by team members on an individual basis. Nonetheless, visible senior management support was important to maintain morale, as indicated by one internal memorandum: 'I am concerned that the initiative should not be stifled by internal disputes regarding accountability and responsibility. It is imperative that this new project is not hampered by demarcation disputes, professional sniping and the sort of paranoia which has greeted innovatory moves in the past.'

For the care managers it seemed that the best way to legitimate their role and to resolve operational difficulties was to provide effective services to older people and their carers, but this of course required them to have the necessary procedures and working arrangements in place. These included systems of assessment, recording, budgeting, arranging services and making payments for services recruited outside the department. Initial discussions with staff from the Personal Social Services Research Unit (PSSRU) and Kent Social Services Department had taken place with frontline staff to provide information and give them the opportunity to discuss concerns, although this work had to be repeated by the care managers themselves in explaining their work and in raising referrals.

### Operational procedures and budgetary accountability

Inevitably the establishment of a new style of service which, however sensitively managed, effectively challenges the established patterns of provision and procedures will lead to turf disputes and experience certain teething difficulties. However, the most problematic issue which faced the establishment of the scheme was to agree procedures for the use of a devolved budget, despite the fact the initiative was building upon the experience of other local authorities.

At the time, the idea of devolving substantial budgets to the level of the frontline social worker was not common in social services departments and there was some disquiet both within social services and in other departments of the local authority. Administrators saw it as necessary for such a new service to fit into existing patterns of organisation, service provision and procedures. From the perspective of some social services managers and the treasurers department there was a risk of loss of financial control, and legal officers expressed concern about risk when expenditure was to be incurred in purchasing services outside the authority. The personnel department had concerns about individuals contracted to provide services for older people and their precise legal relationship with the local authority. The range of concerns which had to be considered in series of negotiations were summarised thus by a senior manager close to the scheme:

> Devolved budgets, a very simple term for a complex procedure. Delegation of power, empowering front line staff, local decision making may seem an unachievable Utopia. It doesn't have to be but many people have to go through painful change to get there, some most reluctantly.

> Devolved budgeting soon starts to sound pretty threatening from a traditionalist standpoint. Managers who have stretched the depths of their own resources to cope with budget ceilings, economic constraint and increasing demands have great difficulty in giving up the task to social workers who at the best of times are rarely seen as committed and competent administrators.

> Personnel officers fully conversant with the content of green and purple books are reluctant to agree the need for the appointment of 'maverick' staff, with conditions of service and tasks undertaken designed by social workers which cannot be compared to anything in their learned texts.

> Legal services need to be reassured that flexibility of approach does not result in a greater risk to the Council.

> Finance department audit staff have difficulty in accepting shifts in financial accountability from experienced time served systems to social workers, of all people. Here to agree about the nature of unit costs was fundamental particularly since it involved asking questions never asked before.

Hence, despite the authority having a clear commitment to the scheme, establishing suitable procedures to permit flexible use of the budget proved to be a lengthy process of negotiation between different departments of the local authority and would not have proved possible without visible social services senior management commitment. Many existing procedures did not prove appropriate for the new scheme, although there was an expectation that the scheme had to prove that these did not work before arrangements could be set in train to produce new ones. The most difficult decisions in this respect were the means for recruiting and paying people as helpers to individual older people and authorising other budget expenditures and this is discussed in more detail in Chapter 4. The process of experimentation with unsatisfactory procedures was inevitably frustrating and at times demoralising for staff whose main concern was to provide support for vulnerable individuals. For the team members this was managed only by keeping a clear view of the underlying goals and necessary structure and features of the scheme. The development of new operational procedures was worked through at assistant director level across local authority departments in conjunction with the scheme team leader. This process took several months, although in the end considerable goodwill was developed towards the scheme by key actors in other departments, particularly those who became closely involved who had absorbed the underlying rationale, and who assisted considerably in the scheme's development.

It became clear that many decisions undertaken in the scheme would be in effect new policy decisions and that for the scheme to succeed it would be continually pressing upon and extending the boundaries of existing systems. The management of this process was both a source of anxiety and concern and also very stimulating. The skilful and alert way in which this was handled by the team leader was an important contribution to the positive developments of the scheme.

Thus the experience of the scheme indicates clearly how the setting up of a care management service requires action not just at the practice level but also at the managerial level. It was only too clear that for the care management service to provide effective service *content* for older people and their carers it had to work in an appropriate facilitating *context*. Failure to address the needs of the service on these different levels would have meant that key elements of the scheme, such as flexibility, would have been lost to procedural requirements and the approach distorted from its original purpose.

## *Underlying attitudes and experiences*

The concerns of a number of different interests in the organisation reflected the scheme's perceived impact either upon day-to-day practice or upon operation of time honoured procedures. On occasions it seemed that this reflected broader underlying attitudes to the care of older people, such as the view that such specialised services were unnecessary for this service user group or that frail older people should not be allowed to live alone in the community because of the risk factors involved. Previous experience of innovations can also be influential and sometimes a new service can be seen in the light of previous unsuccessful projects. Certainly, at times in the early phase, the care managers felt themselves to have been tested out with particularly difficult referrals until such time as the scheme was accepted.

## Undertaking the core tasks of care management

The core tasks of care management are described below under the standard headings commonly employed (Steinberg and Carter, 1983; SSI/SWSG, 1991a,b).

## Case-finding and screening

As has been discussed elsewhere (Challis and Davies, 1986; Davies and Challis, 1986), the processes of case-finding and screening contribute to vertical target efficiency and horizontal target efficiency, both indicators of how well a service is meeting the needs of those for whom its is designed. The first relates to whether the service is accessible to those for whom it is designed and the second to the extent to which those who actually receive the service are those for whom it was designed. Unlike care management services in the USA, of course, there was no financial eligibility screening but only of levels of need.

The scheme, like many care management programmes, was specifically targeted at a sub-group of older people, those who face extreme difficulties in coping at home, despite the input of services, and whose needs are at a level where entry to residential, nursing home, or long-term hospital care is a realistic consideration. This was therefore a specialism within the more general area of the provision of care to older people. Care management can be seen as having a particular role within the more general spectrum of services for vulnerable older people, for whom a limited, prescribed range of services was insufficient.

For targeting purposes, the criteria of need for residential care were discussed in detail with the catchment area district social work team and definitions of this population were provided, based upon available guidelines. Nonetheless, it was recognised that any such definition required the exercise of considerable judgement, and screening was at first undertaken by senior staff in that team prior to referral to the care management service. The care management team leader would again screen referrals prior to their allocation to one of the care managers. Thus initially, referrals were directed through the social services department area teams covering the districts in which the scheme was operating. This provided a reasonably effective mechanism for screening referrals. Care managers' attendance at allocation meetings led to the speedier identification of suitable cases and on occasions the initial assessment of an apparently highly suitable case would be undertaken by them, rather than the teams. It proved important to invest in the process of communicating the nature of suitable cases to referral agents and convince them of the value of the innovation before actively taking on cases. This was designed to protect the scheme from being forced in the first instance to accept unsuitable cases (Seidl et al., 1983). Figure 3.1 shows the referral and screening process for both hospital and community based teams. As can be seen, initial eligibility judgements for care management were undertaken by the teams who would decide whether the person was eligible for the care management service, should be directly referred to domiciliary services or whether their care would be coordinated as the responsibility of the respective team. A small proportion of cases would be referred to the care management service, identified on the basis of their perceived level of need and risk. It is quite helpful to see this differentiation

**Figure 3.1**
*The referral and screening process*

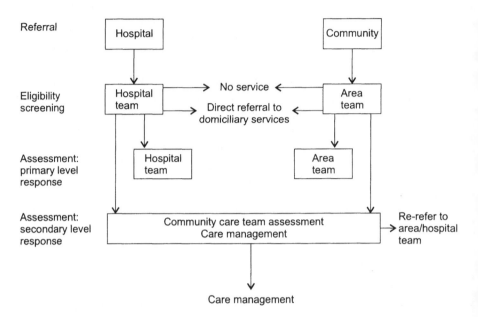

in terms of the teams representing a primary level response, and the care management service as a secondary level response (Challis et al., 1998a).

Once the service became known in the locality and referrals came specifically for the service, initial screening by care managers became more common. General practitioners and community nurses were frequently the source of these. One aspect of case-finding, described as a specific task in the Department of Health guidelines on care management (SSI/SWSG, 1991a,b) is that of publicising the service. In setting up the new service contacts had been established with voluntary organisations, general practitioners and community nurses but these did not become an important source of referrals until the service had been visibly operating in the locality for about six to nine months. Of course, some cases within the target population are not recipients of service and were therefore unknown to providers such as area teams. There were three of these groups for whom the scheme appeared particularly appropriate and whose uptake of services it increased. These were firstly those where the majority of care was provided by stressed informal carers, those who were by and large too frail for much existing social service provision, and those who tended to refuse to accept traditional services, perhaps due to factors such as a psychiatric disorder.

During the time of monitoring the scheme, 101 cases were referred and accepted as appropriate. Of these referrals, many of which had been processed through the area team, 40 per cent were from NHS sources, particularly general practitioners, hospitals and community nurses, and 31 per cent were from social services, family, friends or neighbours. They were a frail group, with an average age of 81, and most were female. Over two-thirds had an identifiable informal carer and two-thirds of these carers were considered to be suffering from stress. Incontinence and confusion were problems for one third of the cases, whilst immobility and risk of falling affected a higher proportion. Most required help with key activities of daily living and all with household chores. Further details on the characteristics of these individuals are provided in Chapter 6.

*Assessment*

A comprehensive assessment was central to the scheme's aim of creating individual, flexible packages of care which were responsive to changes in need. It was evident, as noted before (Challis and Davies, 1985, 1986), that the greater flexibility of response given to the fieldworkers provided an incentive for more detailed assessments, since it was possible to respond to the needs which were identified. The breadth of vision demanded in this more comprehensive approach to assessment avoids the narrow vision of service-oriented assessments, which are all too frequent in care of older people (Goldberg and Connelly, 1982). The assessment was aided by a detailed structured assessment form which was completed within the space of the first few visits and a monitoring chart which detailed an older person's daily activities and support over a usual week (Challis and Chesterman, 1985).

The assessment took into account the circumstances of the older person, their carers, and any services that were involved. Box 3.4 summarises some of the key aspects of the assessment process. Assessment covered the older person's physical and mental health, their attitude and outlook, and environmental and social circumstances, as well as their views of their most pressing problems and desired solutions. The care manager could be involved in balancing the differing and potentially conflicting perceptions and demands of the older person and an informal carer. Equally, the role of other agencies had to be considered, to prevent the overloading of any one service provider, or the provision of care by several different sources in an uncoordinated fashion. This detailed approach to assessment required a variety of skills and knowledge and medical, nursing and therapy staff were often involved in contributing to a valid overall picture of the older person.

Two other elements were seen as crucial to effective assessment: the evaluation of risk and the identification of retained abilities or strengths (Kivnick, 1991). Perceptions of what was tolerable differed between families, other agencies and indeed social services staff themselves. The care manager was required to hold a clear conception of what constituted acceptable risk for a given individual and work to achieve a balance between the views of others

UNIVERSITY OF WINCHESTER
LIBRARY

---

**Box 3.4**

*Aspects of the assessment process*

**Comprehensiveness**

1. Physical, material, emotional and social circumstances of older person.
2. Difficulties and stresses of informal carers.
3. Older person's and carer's perceptions of needs and solutions.
4. Contribution of other services.
5. Use skills of other professionals — medical, physiotherapy, etc.

**Problem-oriented**

1. Not based in narrow limits of one service or existing pattern of provision; breadth of vision of the care managers.

**Needs, strengths and obstacles**

1. Identify remaining skills and motivations and character.
2. Strength of existing networks and relationships.
3. Identify obstacles and barriers to be overcome: e.g. service patterns, reluctance of client/carer to receive services, conflicts.

---

and the rights of the older person. This could be particularly important with those individuals suffering from dementia, where the field worker might have to adopt a role which is protective of the individual older person's residual skill and abilities (Wasser, 1971). All too often the focus of assessment is on the negative aspects of deficits acquired by the older person. However, an effective care plan could only be built upon abilities and skills, which could be maintained and developed by appropriate services. Well-meaning intentions could undermine an individual's independence where, for example, it may be quicker for an outsider to cook a meal or dress an older person, rather than encouraging that person to do as much as possible for themselves. Thus, the approach was to find ways of providing care that would safeguard the older person's abilities and interests, and was concerned with identifying needs, strengths and obstacles to effective interventions.

The amount of care manager time spent on an initial assessment ranged from 9.25 hours to 15 hours. This time included face-to-face contact with the older person and their carer, travel time, administration and time spent liaising with other service providers. Of course, in addition to care manager time, there were hidden costs of external assessors, working in parallel with the care manager. Thus, for example in one case the time of the care manager was augmented by nine hours of the time of other social services and health service staff (Challis et al., 1990b). This timing reflects the initial assessment process, prior to the establishment of a care plan. Of course, in long-term care management assessment is more of a continuous process. In much of the literature reference is made to assessment and care management, as if they were parts of a linear process (Beardshaw and Towell, 1990; SSI/SWSG, 1991a,b). This reflects the role of assessment firstly in delimitation of eligibility for care. Subsequently, care management can be seen as one option which, for some cases, can integrate the assessment of needs and the planning, creation and review of individual care packages. Certainly, accurate assessment will determine the adequacy of these other core tasks of care management. However, assessment may be usefully defined as 'a continuous process of identifying problems and determining what should be done about them' (Hoghughi, 1980, p.20). This is shown in Figure 3.2.

**Figure 3.2**
*Assessment*

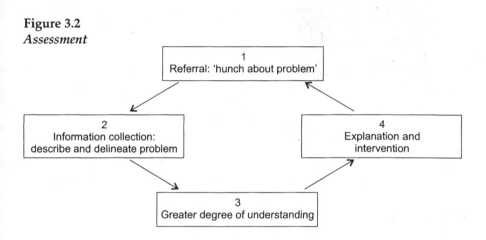

The history of long-term social care, particularly that of older people, is one where the task of assessment has often been performed in a perfunctory and narrow fashion (SSI, 1987). Often, what has been described as assessment has been concerned rather more with a judgement of eligibility for a particular service. Hence, it is important to distinguish between the different features of assessment within the care management process:

- The eligibility screening judgement.
- Initial assessment and problem specification.
- Re-assessment and re-evaluation of the initial formulation.

Given this continuing role of assessment through the care management process, one of the features of this service was the way in which all these different components were lodged with one person, the scheme care managers.

### Care planning and organising services

Based on the detailed assessment, and taking into account the choices expressed by the older person and their carers, an individual care plan was devised to meet the identified needs. The approach to care planning is shown in Box 3.5. This approach overcomes the more common response of a hastily constructed and uncoordinated package developed in response to different demands through time. Not uncommonly, the package of care consisted of mobilising and reorganising the input of existing services, whose individual arrangements may seem quite rational, but whose collective input may not at all be the best use of resources for the older person. This often required patient, tactful negotiations to achieve economical use of existing resources since other statutory services could be reluctant to disrupt their programmes of work to adapt to the needs of a particular older person. Neighbours, family and friends would sometimes prefer not to commit themselves to undertaking certain activities at particular times of day, but may prefer to call on a purely ad hoc basis, which rendered it difficult to include them as part of a regular pattern of care. Fine judgements were required about when and how it was necessary to intervene in family support to improve the quality of care without interfering unreasonably in the lives and relationships of others. On occasions a considerable amount of work was required to assist some reluctant older people or families to receive the necessary level of help and to introduce it at a pace which was acceptable.

The steps involved in moving from the assessment to the construction and implementation of a care package followed a basic hierarchy of need. Thus, ensuring warmth, safety, nutritional and personal care needs were inevitably the primary goals. The pace at which this could be achieved depended on individual circumstances and it was only feasible to attempt higher goals once basic help had been introduced in an acceptable way and proved to be appropriate. Although in a few cases progressing beyond the meeting of very extensive basic needs was difficult, in most situations the personal help and stimulation offered was also designed to improve the older person's morale and quality of life. The decision process thus involved identifying what was to be done, at what pace, in what quantities and in what ways, set against a backcloth of risk evaluation.

New forms of help were developed using the budget under the fieldworkers' control. In common with the Kent scheme people were required who could work flexibly at different times throughout the day to undertake a

---

**Box 3.5**
*Aspects of the care planning process*

**Construct individual care plans based on detailed information**

1. Prioritise *type* of intervention based on hierarchy of need.
2. Identify appropriate *pace* and *level* of intervention.
3. Identify appropriate *way*, involving older person and carer, in which help should be introduced.
4. Identify *level* of acceptable risk.

wide variety of tasks that do not often fall within the remit of traditional services. Building on the Kent experience, Gateshead employed a flexible group of staff with full conditions of service, paid on a sessional basis. These people became known as 'helpers'. The scheme set out to find people with a caring motivation who showed the ability to approach care in the flexible way a new service required. A number of helpers were recruited through publicity with local voluntary groups, press advertising and leaflets displayed in libraries, post offices and shops. In time, the networks of existing helpers proved to be fruitful.

Careful interviews were undertaken with each potential helper, not only to judge their suitability but also to identify characteristics, which might provide the basis for subsequent matching with an older person. Most helpers were female, partly because of the preferences of older people, mainly women themselves, but also because of the nature of the work. Most, three-quarters, were between 31 and 50 years, reflecting a preference for maturer people when coping with the types of tasks required and the vulnerability of many older people. Most, 87 per cent were married and over two-thirds had children under seventeen living at home. In the Kent scheme a higher proportion of older helpers were recruited (Quereshi et al., 1989). Helpers were recruited through adverts in newspapers (31 per cent), another helper (23 per cent) and from adverts in libraries or shops (15 per cent). Over a quarter had part-time work in addition to their work for the scheme. On average helpers worked visiting older people for about ten hours per week.

Every attempt was made to match available helpers to the needs of particular older people. Obviously location and the availability of the potential helper were important in the first instance. Thus, the scheme aimed to encourage the involvement of members of the local community with its older residents. In practical terms, help offered to frail older people had to be capable of responding in emergencies and be reliable in bad weather. However, personality and skills were also important factors. For example, a helper could live near and have the time available to help a confused person get ready in the morning, but might find herself unable to cope with the unpredictability of such a person's care needs. Again, for some older people with mobility problems, knowledge of lifting techniques could be important. In matching, the aim was to make possible a relationship that would give stimulation and meet the social needs of the older person as well as providing basic care. Matching of workload also proved important so that capable helpers did not only experience the least rewarding older people and become overburdened. Training was provided for helpers in areas such as recognition of problems and lifting. A new helper was always introduced to an older person by the care manager, who would discuss the tasks required and any possible difficulties. The helper would then be issued with a contract specifying days, times and tasks to be undertaken. This contract was updated every time there was a permanent change in visiting, and was seen as important in setting boundaries to helpers' involvement, in avoiding excess burden, and in legitimising their role.

The tasks which helpers undertook were wide-ranging, and some of the more common activities are noted in Table 3.1.

The data presented in Table 3.1 are based upon the workload of 68 helpers over a four-week period, representing 272 helper weeks in all. As can be seen a considerable amount of activity involved ensuring adequate diet and meal preparation, the provision of personal care, help with maintaining continence, the provision of social support, and assisting people with dementia in reassurance and reality orientation. Helpers undertook other therapeutic activities less frequently, such as teaching older people skills such as dressing and working independently following a stroke under the supervision of a physiotherapist. Activities not noted here include tasks helpers undertook beyond what was specified in their contract, such as taking the older person on outings. The demands upon the care manager, in using helpers to both fill care gaps and to respond more appropriately to choice, involved effecting the entry of this additional help, ensuring it fitted with the pre-existing care network, renegotiating existing levels of care, and providing support and guidance to the helpers.

**Table 3.1**

*Tasks undertaken by helpers: social care scheme*

| Task | Percentage[a] |
|---|---|
| Light housework | 57 |
| Shopping for daily or weekly needs | 52 |
| Washing soiled items | 22 |
| Make meals in client's home | 73 |
| Prepare snack or hot drink | 66 |
| Take meal from own home to client | 34 |
| Clear away stale food | 50 |
| Monitor amount client has eaten/drunk | 22 |
| Help with heating system (gas, electric, central heating) | 34 |
| Help with getting up and going to bed | 67 |
| Help with dressing and undressing | 65 |
| Brush or comb hair | 55 |
| Help with washing older person | 34 |
| Help to use toilet or commode | 41 |
| Clean or empty commode, bottle or bedpan | 57 |
| Change/dispose of incontinence pads/sheets | 21 |
| Give/check tablets/medication | 66 |
| Companionship and stimulation | 88 |
| Reality orientation | 35 |
| Provide reassurance if client agitated | 25 |

a Based on 4 week period by 68 helpers, percentage of 272 weeks that task was done.

Although helpers were the main cost to the budget, other activities were also developed. It became evident early on that a number of older people were neglecting their diet. Meals-on-wheels were not sufficient as they were neither tempting nor offered encouragement to eat. A number of older people were also artificially housebound due to lack of transport, they had no escort, or had no acceptable place to go. To combat these problems, small day care groups were established in several helpers' homes, based around a meal-time. These groups proved to be of considerable value from the point of view of increasing social outlets, making new relationships, and stimulating appetite. At other times the budget was used to purchase vacuum-packed meals that merely required re-heating. These offered a wider choice of menu, a choice of time to eat and provided a standby for holidays, periods of bad weather or other emergencies. The budget was also used to buy aids, either for short-term loan until they could be obtained from the usual sources, or to provide items not usually available. These items included automatic kettles or smoke alarms for use by people with dementia, oil-filled radiators to supplement inadequate heating and special flasks for hot drinks that were easy to use for those with arthritis. Handicrafts for rehabilitative and recreational purposes, which were not normally available, were also purchased.

Table 3.2 provides a summary of the services that care managers either liaised with or used most frequently in order to develop a care plan. It can be seen that contact with a range of health service providers was particularly important. The general practitioner was noted in nearly two-thirds of reviews, community nurses in 39 per cent, bathing aides in 29 per cent, and chiropody in 26 per cent. The central role of the home help service and the scheme helpers, cited in 80 per cent and 92 per cent of reviews respectively, is clearly evident, particularly given that the first review took place a month after referral when the full package of care would not necessarily have been established for all cases. An occupational therapist was often involved in the assessment and a wide range of aids was used. The provision of meals was also noted in more than half of the case reviews. Hence, it can be seen that care managers had to organise a number of services for each older person. The median number of services received was five, with 11 per cent of older people receiving two or less services and 17 per cent receiving seven or more services.

Case review data also provided a summary of the care problems dealt with by care managers over a one-year period for 101 cases.

Table 3.3 indicates that the main problems tackled in care plans were those arising from functional disabilities, particularly in the areas of personal care, rising and retiring and household care. Also important were ill health, family stress, and isolation and loneliness of the older person. Although confusional states were only noted in 10 per cent of the reviews, factors associated with this condition were more commonly cited. These included difficulties in managing financial affairs, difficulties with activities of daily living and family stress. Indeed, work supporting families and dealing with conflict in relationships

**Table 3.2**
*Resources used by care managers: social care scheme*

| Service | Percentage of reviews |
|---|---|
| General practitioner | 64 |
| Community nurse | 39 |
| Bath attendant | 29 |
| Chiropody | 26 |
| Geriatric hospital/outpatients department | 9 |
| Other hospital/outpatients department | 23 |
| Home help | 80 |
| Paid helper (social care scheme) | 92 |
| Meals | 54 |
| Social clubs/outings | 22 |
| Street wardens | 10 |
| SSD telephone | 9 |
| Occupational therapy | 23 |
| Aids for mobility | 41 |
| Aids for toileting | 33 |
| Aids for bathing | 28 |
| Aids for household use | 33 |
| Aids for hearing | 10 |
| Housing department | 14 |
| Social security | 9 |

**Table 3.3**
*Client problems tackled: social care scheme*

| Client problem tackled | Percentage of reviews | Most important problem (%) |
|---|---|---|
| Physical disability/illness | 34 | 12 |
| Visual difficulties | 11 | 2 |
| Hearing difficulties | 11 | 1 |
| Incontinence | 10 | 1 |
| Difficulties arising a.m./p.m. | 25 | 5 |
| Personal care problems | 39 | 12 |
| Daily household problems | 46 | 13 |
| Weekly household problems | 20 | 2 |
| Psychological/emotional problems | 18 | 7 |
| Confusional states | 10 | 3 |
| Social isolation/loneliness | 45 | 12 |
| Family relations problems | 41 | 17 |
| Accommodation problems | 17 | 5 |
| Managing affairs problems | 11 | 0 |

was identified as the most important problem across the reviews, and therefore of the care managers' workload.

*Monitoring and reviewing care*

Neither the process of assessment nor of care planning can be considered as one-off activities. They are dynamic and continuously build on the progress of earlier work and require responses to changing circumstances and previously concealed problems. In the provision of intensive care at home, forming a tailor-made package of support devised through the care manager's assessment with control over budgetary resources requires close monitoring. This was of course more complex than simply monitoring an individual service. The usual pattern of intervention was one of long-term monitoring, regular adjustments of service, and periodic, short-term, direct involvement where circumstances dictated. This could take the form of direct work with an older person, in responding to psychological or emotional needs, or involve work with the carers in tackling the problems and strains that they encountered. Intervention could also be more indirect, working through helpers and other service providers and training them in particular approaches such as reality orientation. A considerable amount of time was spent in supporting helpers, both individually and in groups. Much effort was spent upon ensuring effective communications to ensure understanding and coordination in the care network of each older person. Without this, breakdown in the pattern of care could too easily occur. The use of monitoring charts and notebooks left in the older person's house were further aids to good communication. The role of the care manager was to assess the effectiveness of the inputs, including those of the helpers, to identify potential problems or mismatches and to obtain a smoothly functioning team approach. As part of the recording system, formal case reviews were completed at four-monthly intervals, identifying problems encountered, the present situation, changes to be aimed for over the next period, intervention plans and contacts with agencies. Comparison of reviews over time could give a longer view and put into perspective day-to-day events (Challis and Chesterman, 1985, 1986).

Table 3.4 summarises the main activities undertaken based upon the frequency with which a particular activity occurred in the reviews. It can be seen that close monitoring of the well-being of older people and the adequacy of the care provided was the most frequently undertaken activity, occurring in 90 per cent of reviews. Providing general support to the older person (60 per cent), their family (43 per cent) and scheme helpers (72 per cent) was another frequently noted area of work. Assessment and reassessment were activities undertaken in 46 per cent of reviews indicating how assessment cannot be seen as a single 'event' in care management, but as part of a recurrent process. This was the activity seen as most important across the reviews. The activities of mobilising and coordinating resources were frequently undertaken, noted

**Table 3.4**
*Care managers' activities: social care scheme*

| Care manager activities | Percentage of reviews | Most important activity (%) |
|---|---|---|
| Assessment/re-assessment | 46 | 26 |
| Information/advice | 22 | 2 |
| Mobilising resources | 66 | 12 |
| Coordinating resources | 65 | 8 |
| Check-up/review visits | 90 | 6 |
| Facilitating problem-solving/decision-making | 29 | 12 |
| Sustaining/nurturing client | 60 | 9 |
| Sustaining/nurturing family/informal carers | 43 | 8 |
| Sustaining/nurturing helpers | 72 | 13 |
| Advocacy | 14 | 4 |

in about two-thirds of the reviews. Activities involving helping older people to identify and choose between solutions to problems were noted in nearly one third of reviews. This, coupled with the proportion of activity devoted to a range of support activities indicates how this form of care management involved substantially more than the organisation and processing of services (SSI, 1997).

The argument in favour of intensive care management is that it constitutes an integrated investment in a series of activities — assessment, service coordination, monitoring and support of older people and their carers, and continuity of care — to provide more effective and efficient support that would otherwise be the case. One indicator of the extent to which this investment of resource in care management was appropriate is the consistency of the proportion of costs attributable to care management. In the Gateshead social care scheme care management costs were 18 per cent of social services and 9 per cent of the joint social services and NHS costs (Challis et al., 1990b). These proportions are similar to the costs for the health and social care scheme and the Darlington study (Challis et al., 1990b, 1995). These proportions are shown in Table 3.5.

**Table 3.5**
*The proportion of costs attributable to care management*

| | SSD | SSD and NHS |
|---|---|---|
| Gateshead social care | 18% | 9% |
| Gateshead health and social care | 17% | 11% |
| Darlington | 14% | 10% |

Thus, overall, it can be seen that the care managers were required to undertake a considerable amount of both indirect work, coordinating and liaising with others, and direct face-to-face work in assessing, helping older people to make crucial decisions and providing support to them, their carers and other service providers.

## Case closure

The focus of the care managers' work was to enable frail older people to remain at home as an alternative to residential or nursing home care, whenever that was their wish. However, at times they had to be responsible for evaluating the appropriate balance between the wishes of older people, the levels of risk that this entailed and the pressures experienced by their carers. For some individuals it was the case that their interests were better met in a residential setting and the care manager was responsible for providing help in effecting this decision and enabling the older person and their carers to manage the transition. Of course, at the time of the social care study, the residential care sector was one where a significant proportion of placements were in local authority provision, and where subsequent reviews would be undertaken as a responsibility of the home. Hence, for most cases the care managers were able to close cases once the process of placement and management of the transition had been accomplished. This meant that even through time the main focus of their activity could be the support and maintenance of people in their own homes, rather than an increasing proportion of their time being spent upon review of individuals in residential settings. This is important in maintaining programme integrity and avoiding distortions, which have been observed in other programmes (Challis, 1994a). Thus, case closure would occur in nearly all cases following a long-term care placement.

## Supervision and managing the care management service

We have so far described the ways in which the core tasks of care management were undertaken in the social care scheme. Earlier in the chapter it was noted how care management can be seen as a multi-level response, involving care level activities and service development, a distinction described as being between care management practice and care management systems (O'Connor, 1988). The care management team was small and had its own management structure, linking into the mainstream management processes at a high level. Hence, day-to-day management, strategy and service development were the responsibility of the team leader. The range of responsibilities at that time was probably broader than would have been the norm within most agencies, since it covered the whole range of activities of staff supervision, budget management, service planning and development and carrying a small caseload. This required the team manager to look simultaneously in the direction of implementation and content of practice and also at a system level evaluating caseload mix, budget allocations and quality assurance. An innovatory scheme, for its survival and development, required an effective product champion and this proved to be a crucial role from its inception. Indeed, in the absence of a member of staff with this specific responsibility it is likely that the scheme would not have developed as effectively. Service development involved effectively locating aspects of policy formulation and development with the immediate management of care managers, as has occurred in other service developments (Raiff and Shore, 1993). Formal supervision of staff was undertaken on a monthly basis and although inevitably individual case and practice focused, also led to discussions about service development. This was made feasible by the substantial devolved budget, which was at the discretion of the team manager.

In performing supervisory, managerial and quality assurance responsibilities the team manager was aided by the presence of the team's own information system. This consisted of a structured assessment document, regular case reviews undertaken at least on a four-monthly basis for each older person, and weekly costings based upon all social services inputs to each case. Hence, for individual supervision it was possible to review changes in needs, patterns of response, and strategies of care employed, so as to consider issues of quality and effectiveness. At a more general level, it was possible to consider casemix for the scheme as a whole and expenditure trends on a reliable basis. This information system, which permitted monitoring of the key question 'who gets what with what outcomes?' is described in more detail in Challis and Chesterman (1985, 1986). It provided the data about activities and patterns of contact by care managers, described earlier in this chapter. During the phase of monitoring the social care scheme, 101 older people were supported and over a year these service users could have generated four case reviews each. Due to institutionalisation and death, there were 357 case reviews completed. This case review material has provided a convenient summary of the activities which constituted the care managers' workload, and, suitably aggregated, could form the basis for performance measures, particularly when combined with cost and assessment information.

Box 3.6 shows some of the key roles and tasks involved in the management of care management. There are five broad areas identified: service management, quality assurance, staff supervision, within agency coordination, and between agency coordination. Service management involved both the administration and financial management of the care management service. It also involved evaluating the implications of expenditure patterns for the management group. Quality assurance required the maintenance and use of the information system and close monitoring of the eligibility and targeting criteria. This required examination of assessment processes and liaison with key referral agents within the social services department. It also involved ensuring the

---

**Box 3.6**
*The management of care management: roles and tasks*

**Management of the service**

Administration and financial management of the service.

Day-to-day administration of the service.

Project cost implications of care packages for immediate budget planning.

**Quality assurance**

Develop, maintain and appropriately use information systems.

Monitor eligibility and targeting criteria.

Ensure assessments and care plans are completed in good time.

Ensure service plans are appropriate.

Check the satisfaction of older people and carers.

Monitor the costs of care packages.

**Staff supervision**

Support for care managers and skill development.

Identify and implement training needs.

Establish lateral supervision through peer review and analysis of case histories.

**Coordination within agency**

Ensure smooth functioning of operational systems such as finance, contracting and
    purchasing.

Membership of relevant cross-departmental working groups.

**Collaboration between agencies**

Contribute to planning and development of services.

Improve information flow and coordination between service providers.

Membership of inter-agency liaison group.

Sources: Steinberg and Carter (1983); Kendig et al. (1992); Challis et al. (1995).

---

timely completion of assessments and care plans and ensuring that service allocations were appropriate, both in terms of resource relevance and cost. Another important activity was ensuring the mechanisms were in place to check that older people and their carers were satisfied with the care they received. This could involve ensuring care managers undertook regular reviews, or the team leader visiting certain cases to ascertain that arrangements were appropriate. Ensuring that patterns of cost were equitably distributed between broadly similar cases was another important task.

Staff supervision had several different facets. Firstly, it involved providing support and guidance to the care managers and enabling them to expand and employ new skills. The role of care manager, with freedom to allocate resources and develop services, was a new one and staff at times would require their horizons lifting, so as to approach problems in new ways. In the absence of this, experience in the US indicates that even where care managers have access to flexible resources care plans may still be over predictable (Schneider, 1989; Kane, 1990). Inevitably in large bureaucratic organisations the use of unconventional strategies in providing care could at times provoke resistance from other sections of the department. This was particularly evident in the support of some older people with confusional states described later in Chapter 5. In encouraging service development there was an important management role in providing support to care managers, so that they could work in a more creative fashion, at times being the care managers' care manager (Raiff and Shore, 1993). Sometimes this would identify particular training needs, such as care of older people with dementia. In order to spread lessons from new forms of good practice, a deliberate process of joint supervisory activity was established whereby individual, novel strategies of care were shared. This was particularly important in a phase when the new service was trying to establish itself, with its own norms and practices, which were not always fully consonant with those of the host agency. The newness of the service, requiring different operational systems for the management of budgets, external purchasing and contracting, required the team leader to liaise on a regular basis with a number of other departments within the authority, and to participate in cross-departmental working groups.

It was also important for the management of the scheme to feed into inter-agency planning groups, since the advent of a new form of social care provision for older people required at times a re-negotiation of boundaries with community health services. Later, as the service developed and particular shortfalls, such as health service input into the assessment process, were identified, this led to the development of a joint pilot scheme, with an additional nurse care manager and medical assessor within the team — the health and social care scheme. This extension to the original social care scheme is described in Chapter 9.

# 4 The Role of Helpers and their Experience of the Scheme

This chapter is concerned with the experience of helpers in the scheme. Chapter 3 described how helpers were an important means for the care managers to provide more individually tailored services and to fill gaps in care. This chapter considers such factors as the balance of motivations and rewards of those involved in part-time activities, which blur the boundaries of traditional voluntary activity and paid part-time work.

The data upon which the present chapter is based has been drawn from two sources. Most of the information is derived from interviews with a group of 119 helpers. At the time of interview they had been working for the scheme between anything from a few weeks to over two years. A second source of information was a survey of the range and frequency of the tasks undertaken by helpers over a four-week time period. Based upon 68 helpers, this provided information for 272 weeks in all and gave a picture of the usual range of care tasks undertaken in the social care scheme.

The chapter begins by describing the helpers, their previous experience and their reasons for joining the scheme. The next section looks at the range of care tasks undertaken, including their initial introduction to the older person, the quantity and nature of the tasks they undertook, their relationship with the older person and informal carers, the support they received from the care managers and other helpers, their contact with workers from other agencies, and the degree to which it led to further activity outside the scheme. The helpers' role, satisfactions and drawbacks of the work are considered and the relationship between the initial motivations of helpers and the rewards they received is examined, and also the factors which led to helpers leaving the scheme (Qureshi et al., 1989).

## The helpers' backgrounds and experience

Some three-quarters of the helpers were aged between 31 and 50 (Table 4.1). It is noteworthy that only one helper was aged under 21, and only two aged over 60. The latter was a direct result of the local authority policy by which helpers could only receive an income as a paid employee, so could obtain no fee above pensionable age. All but two of the helpers were female. This probably reflects a view amongst the local male population that the work was essentially 'women's work', although it must not be forgotten that most of the older people were themselves female, for whom a woman carer was often preferable.

**Table 4.1**

*Age range of the helpers*

| Age | % |
|-----|---|
| 18-20 | 1 |
| 21-30 | 8 |
| 31-40 | 44 |
| 41-50 | 30 |
| 51-60 | 15 |
| 61 and over | 2 |

Number of helpers = 119

Some of the financial, housing and social circumstances of the helpers are summarised in Table 4.2. It can be seen that the vast majority were married, and over two-thirds had children under 17 living at home. One in three was a housewife and one in four in another caring occupation at the time of recruitment. A quarter of helpers were located in council rented property and most of the remainder were owner occupiers.

**Table 4.2**

*Characteristics of the helpers*

| Characteristic | % |
|----------------|---|
| Married | 87 |
| Children under 17 at home | 69 |
| *Usual occupation:* | |
|   housewife | 35 |
|   other caring occupation | 23 |
|   other | 42 |
| *Type of housing:* | |
|   owner occupier | 68 |
|   council rented | 25 |
|   private rented | 7 |
| *Financial circumstances of helpers and families during scheme:* | |
|   received state benefit throughout | 18 |
|   received state benefit part of time | 13 |
| *Benefit received by helper:* | |
|   unemployment benefit | 11 |
|   supplementary benefit | 8 |
|   widow's pension | 5 |

Number of helpers = 119

Regarding the financial circumstances of helpers and their families, 18 per cent received state benefit throughout, and 13 per cent for part of the time that they worked for the scheme. The main types of benefit received were unemployment benefit (11 per cent), supplementary benefit (8 per cent) and widow's pension (5 per cent). For one in five, the receipt of state benefit limited their earnings through the scheme, and they experienced problems with the benefit or tax authorities.

### Recruitment and previous experience

The ways in which helpers were recruited for the scheme are shown in Table 4.3. The main methods of recruitment were through newspaper advertising (31 per cent), through another helper (23 per cent) and from advertising in a library or shop (15 per cent). The latter was the main method of recruitment in the early stages of the scheme, whilst newspaper advertising was used rather more once the scheme had become established, and those found through another helper also increased. Nearly one half of the helpers interviewed had already worked for the scheme for at least one year.

**Table 4.3**
*Methods of recruiting helpers over time*

| Method | Recruitment in first year | Recruitment in second year | Subsequent recruitment | All |
|---|---|---|---|---|
| | % | % | % | % |
| Older person's informal network | 7 | 5 | 0 | 4 |
| Advert in library/shop | 30 | 5 | 10 | 15 |
| Advert in newspaper | 22 | 35 | 36 | 31 |
| Voluntary organisation | 3 | 8 | 8 | 6 |
| Another helper | 15 | 30 | 23 | 23 |
| Already caring for older person | 3 | 0 | 5 | 3 |
| Other | 20 | 17 | 18 | 18 |
| Number of helpers | 40 | 40 | 39 | 119 |

Although very few of the helpers were in full-time employment in addition to their work for the scheme, over a quarter had a part-time job. Unsurprisingly, the most frequent type of previous caring experience was with relatives, family or neighbours (90 per cent). Although only a few helpers were trained nurses, in total about one-third had had experience as a nursing auxiliary, in residential homes or day care settings. Thirteen per cent also had previous experience with voluntary organisations.

**Motivation for joining the scheme**

Over half of the helpers (56 per cent) said they were looking for some kind of
job, a somewhat different emphasis from those interviewed in the early phase
of the Kent scheme, which initially attracted a number of unpaid helpers with
more voluntaristic motives, for whom payment was an incidental extra. This
may have been attributable to the Kent scheme being located in a retirement
area, although later differences were less marked (Challis and Davies, 1986).
However, variations in different areas of Kent suggest that there may be important area differences in the characteristics of the helpers attracted. The Gateshead scheme was always presented as a remunerative activity, although not a
conventional job, and may therefore have attracted more people who specifically wanted paid employment. Nevertheless, helpers were simultaneously
likely to say that they were looking for a social activity, a voluntary activity or,
in a few cases, a career-related activity as well as payment. As already noted,
unlike Kent, payment procedures of the local authority excluded those over retirement age.

*General motivational themes*

The themes which helpers themselves spontaneously raised regarding their
motivations are considered below. They fell into nine broad categories, which
overlap to some extent with specific questions based upon the motivations
identified in Qureshi et al. (1983; 1989) and are shown in Table 4.4.

**Table 4.4**
*Specific motivations of helpers*[a]

| Motivation | % |
| --- | --- |
| 1.  To do something useful | 90 |
| 2.  To look after or care for someone | 82 |
| 3.  To help someone in need | 81 |
| 4.  To work with the elderly | 77 |
| 5.  Interest outside the home/separate identity | 68 |
| 6.  To meet people | 60 |
| 7.  To earn some money | 48 |
| 8.  To use skills | 37 |
| 9.  To fill spare time or provide stimulation | 31 |
| 10. Social obligation | 29 |
| 11. Experience for a job or career | 24 |
| 12. To repay help received having had good fortune | 20 |
| 13. To take mind off own worries | 9 |
| 14. Already doing work, but offer of pay was helpful | 3 |
| Number of cases = 119 | |

a  Based upon motivations identified in Qureshi et al. (1983, 1989).

Table 4.4 indicates the helpers' responses to a set of motivational items derived from Qureshi et al. (1989). Most were motivated by the desire to help and undertake useful activity, and about three-quarters were specifically concerned to help older people. Self-development or the application of existing skills were cited by a considerable number of the helpers. Monetary gain was cited by just under a half. The need to fill spare time was noted by about one-third. Aspects of social responsibility were also important for about a quarter of the helpers. One in four were hoping that the scheme would provide them with experience for a future career. About one in ten were trying to achieve a diversion from pressing personal problems, or were engaged in displacement of painful feelings. A handful were simply responding to a request from the team to give more structured help to a person they already visited. Helpers talked much less about these and other sources of motivation, and therefore they have not been pursued.

Interestingly, there were some significant differences between helpers from the inner city and those from the more outlying areas in terms of motivations of social activity, social obligation and altruism. This suggests that, as might be expected, the more instrumental motivations, such as payment, were necessarily more influential in the less affluent area. In comparison with helpers from the Kent scheme (Challis and Davies, 1986; Qureshi et al., 1989), payment was similarly a motivation for less than half, but having time to spare was markedly less influential, suggestive of the differences between the more urban environment of Gateshead and a retirement area.

*Money* As mentioned above, many helpers voiced financial reasons for applying to the scheme. The importance of money is demonstrated by their responses to questions about the relative importance of financial factors. Only about half spontaneously mentioned money as a source of motivation (Table 4.4, 7). In some cases it was a prerequisite for undertaking the work. They needed money and if the scheme had not offered it, they would have felt it necessary to look elsewhere. Sometimes, helpers' or helpers' spouses' existing employment was under threat, or too low paid. Some people disliked their existing jobs but could only transfer to the scheme if it offered money to compensate for their lost wage. Others had particular expenses, such as moving house, so needed extra cash. Thus, about 60 per cent of helpers said that it was either 'very important' or 'quite important' to be able to earn money, whereas only 38 per cent suggested that 'It didn't matter about the money'.

There was evidence, however, of differing reasons between helpers for attaching importance to money. For some where the money motivation was not acute financial need, it was typified as 'an attraction', a welcome financial bonus, or source of some financial independence, rather than as a means of making ends meet. Even when helpers did not need money as a primary reason for doing the work, they often regarded it as an integral part of their commitment to the scheme, and significantly, of the scheme's commitment to them. Indeed some of the helpers least motivated by money were those on state benefit, because they were allowed to keep so little of their earnings. Their only hope, if they needed money, was to look for a regular job that took them beyond eligibility for benefit, and the scheme could not always provide that.

*An accessible job* Nearly one-third of the helpers highlighted the flexibility of the hours of work as a major attraction. Most helpers had family commitments to which they gave priority, and their ideal job was one that did not oblige them to be away from home when their families needed them there. The scheme allowed room for negotiation about the amount of time worked, and when it was worked, and allowed for some variation if necessary.

One helper specified that she would never accept evening or weekend work, because she felt it would impinge on family life. She was most explicit about the benefits of the scheme providing family-based women with a satisfying outlet which, because of the choice over the hours, was realistically available to them. Another helper appreciated being able to do her job in small time segments, slotted conveniently into her own domestic routine:

> I like the flexibility, that you're never away from home for more than an hour at a time.

A few helpers praised the flexible hours because they felt temperamentally unsuited to being tied down to normal working hours, and enjoyed the variation of working different hours on different days.

Helpers mentioned other aspects of working for the scheme which made it accessible to them, as women with family commitments. Several said they valued being able to work so near home, because it minimised the disruption to their domestic routine. Others drew comparisons with alternative part-time, unqualified jobs available to them. Jobs such as shop work, pub work, and cleaning were the most likely alternatives, and they found these both less satisfying as a personal outlet, and less convenient. Some had done auxiliary nursing or other caring jobs which, although they may have liked the work, caused them great difficulties because the shifts, or the overall time commitment of a job with fixed hours, interfered too much with life at home.

There was a price to be paid for this exercise of choice. They could not control whether the scheme offered them work at the times when they wanted it and there was therefore no guaranteed income from one week to the next since it was dependent upon the availability of people needing help. Helpers who stayed with the scheme had to accept the insecurity, as well as the relative autonomy. One helper epitomised the rewards and dilemmas of becoming a helper. She had been working as a cleaner, which gave her little satisfaction, and necessitated working hours that were unsuitable for her family. The scheme offered better hours, was nearer home and was potentially more rewarding, but it meant risking giving up a regular job, and could not guarantee a regular income or continuing employment. Money and an accessible job are the two areas of motivation that can most clearly be regarded as 'instrumental' or goal-directed, and both figured highly, but helpers were rarely single-mindedly instrumental in their approach to the scheme. Most also had other motives. Indeed, if their only motives had appeared to be instrumental, the care managers might well have not accepted them as helpers. It is therefore not surprising that the other sets of motivations identified fall more into the 'expressive' or psychologically oriented range, although the distinctions are far from clear cut in individuals' minds. The following four areas contain clear elements of both.

*Work satisfaction* Although the majority of helpers wanted a relatively formal job, most (59 per cent) said that they would not have taken just 'any job', even with 'comparable pay and conditions'. They wanted work that would be personally satisfying and emotionally rewarding. One helper put it simply:

> I want to be happy going to work, and enjoy what I do.

Many echoed this idea of looking for positive enjoyment from doing work they liked doing.

A sense of usefulness was a major element in job satisfaction, and it is clear from Table 4.4 that the vast majority of helpers responded thus. Many helpers said that they wanted to be socially useful, and providing care for such dependent people was unambiguously useful. In this way, they felt able to play a determining role in the welfare of people who could not manage without their help. As one helper put it, she liked:

> ... being a kind of life-line for the old.

The job satisfaction to be derived from feeling they were doing something so worthwhile was a powerful motivation. Even if helpers were considering jobs other than working for the scheme, they were quite often looking for jobs that they felt might bring similar emotional rewards:

> Before I applied for [scheme], I was looking for a job as a housing warden or a family aide; just something worthwhile, and to do with helping people.

One helper, who had had to leave the scheme because her financial circumstances forced her to find a regular job, was full of regret. She had found the personal caring so rewarding that:

> I liked it — a job against the world.

The attraction of a job which provided satisfaction as well as remuneration is a theme which runs through the interviews and echoes the findings from similar work by Abrams and his colleagues (Bulmer, 1986).

*Self-fulfilment* A strong theme in the interviews was a search for a personal outlet or a new interest, which would bring them a sense of personal fulfilment. This is illustrated by item 5 in Table 4.4. The word 'interesting' crops up again and again as a description of what attracted some helpers to the scheme. Others said they were looking for some stimulation (item 9 in Table 4.4), or liked the idea of the scheme because it 'sounded different', and 'wanted to find out more about it'. Some were very frank about how unstimulating a full-time job as a housewife can be:

> I was really more interested in having something to get me out of a rut, out of the house, doing something different from looking after the family.

This did not imply a lessening of the priority given to their perceived primary role of housewife and family carer:

> I wanted something to get me out of the house a bit, away from the children; but something to fit in with the children and my husband's shifts.

The scheme offered a source of stimulation and satisfaction which was a refreshing change from their own family life, but which most importantly did not threaten or disrupt it. It could extend their interests without entailing any major changes in their lives.

Some helpers were particularly looking for an outlet at this time because they had some time on their hands, typically because their children were at school and growing up, so that mothering was no longer a full-time job; or because a sick or elderly relative for whom they were caring had died or gone into hospital. These helpers wanted something to fill their time, but they did not want just anything. They wanted something that they would find more fulfilling than 'wasting it about the house'.

A few helpers had time available because of early retirement, or redundancy, or because ill health had caused them to give up their regular jobs. They found it important for their morale to find a constructive outlet, 'to use up my energy'. One woman who had been made redundant was quite eloquent about her need for a fulfilling substitute for her last job:

> I applied to keep myself alive. I was unemployed and I have no family. I was looking for work and I thought [scheme] sounded interesting: I needed money, but also, I was very bored being at home all day. I would have done voluntary work if I'd found any, just to get out.

*Social integration* Perhaps an extension of this move to self-fulfilment was some helpers' hope that joining the scheme would help their own integration with the local community. Many said that they not only wanted interesting and satisfying activity, but were also keen that it should 'get me out of the house':

> I felt it [the scheme] was a good thing, helping people, and that it would help me to meet people and get out of the house.

A few helpers had specific integration needs that linked conveniently with their participation in the scheme:

> I was interested in elderly people and had always got on well with them. I had recently moved back into the inner city and I thought it would be a good way of making links locally.

Another helper had not only moved house, but had been suffering some depression and anxiety following a bereavement. She felt that working for the scheme would help her get out and about again, and meet new people. As another helper summed it up:

> There's a lot of people like me, just wanting to work for a few hours in the community.

Nonetheless, it was only a minority of helpers who felt a general need to integrate themselves. Many were already actively involved in their local communities. Perhaps the scheme offered a broadening and deepening of their sense of community participation by formalising and extending their caring role where it already existed, or by offering new openings when helpers felt these were lacking in their lives at that time. This theme of meeting people motivated some two-thirds of helpers (item 6 of Table 4.4).

*A caring identity* The opportunity to become involved semi-professionally in caring was a welcome one for most helpers. One woman said simply:

> I like elderly people, and I enjoy helping people generally.

Many helpers said that they just liked helping people, which is clear from items 2 and 3 in Table 4.4. They were glad of the chance to do it in an organised, legitimate manner.

Sometimes helpers were making up for past lost opportunities to follow a career in caring:

> I've always wanted to do nursing or something like this, i.e. HELPING people. [her emphasis]

Helpers not only often felt a 'natural' attraction to helping people for its own sake (see item 3 in Table 4.4), but they also tended to feel they had the experience and aptitudes which made them suited to the work (see item 8 in Table 4.4). For example, one helper cited as evidence the voluntary neighbouring she was doing:

> I'm used to helping people. I was doing it [before the scheme] without being paid. I thought it [the scheme] was useful work, and something I would be able to do.

Another helper felt she had a lot to offer because:

I'm pretty tolerant of old people.

Several mentioned their informal caring experiences, helping neighbours and caring for relatives; others had more formal experience of being employed in a caring job. They saw the scheme as a vehicle for putting their resulting knowledge and skills to good use. Even those without directly relevant experience felt the scheme offered a recognition of their personal qualities and life experiences.

The scheme's emphasis on relationship and interpersonal qualities, as well as on practical caring, gave helpers scope to express talents that they may not have considered marketable previously. Graham has argued that:

The experience of caring is the medium through which women are accepted into and feel they belong in the social world. It is the medium through which they gain admittance into both the private world of the home and the public world of the labour market. It is through caring in an informal capacity — as mothers, wives, daughters, neighbours, friends — and through formal caring — as nurses, secretaries, cleaners, teachers, social workers — that women can enter their place in society (Graham, 1983, p.30).

The scheme's helpers were self-identified carers, both at home and in the community and often in their existing part-time jobs. For most, the scheme was a development of this identity.

The opportunity to be acknowledged, professionally and financially, for being a person skilled in caring for its own sake, and for being able not only to perform the tasks of tending but also to forge successful caring relationships with individuals, was a major attraction of the scheme.

*Attraction to elderly people* Over two-thirds of helpers said that they wanted to do the work because they just liked older people (item 4 in Table 4.4). One helper put it simply but forcefully:

I LOVE old people, and I want to help them. [her emphasis]

Her grandparents had recently died, and she was longing to bestow her affection on other older people. She shared this kind of 'substitution of affection' motive with other helpers. A basic sympathy with the care needs of the old was essential, but these helpers voiced an exceptional interest in the company of older people. For instance:

I like elderly people very much. I particularly like talking to them about their lives and what the North East used to be like.

Others said that they felt more at ease in the company of older people than that of younger age groups.

Sometimes, helpers had had jobs where they came into contact with older people, but not in a directly caring capacity, as a hospital domestic for example, and had developed an interest in older people's lives which made them want to become more personally involved. Sometimes, hearing about other people's contact with older people had stimulated a latent interest. For these helpers, older people variously offered an easy outlet for their affections, a source of intellectual interest and stimulation, and a rewarding direction for their community service.

*Attraction to the aims of the care scheme* Closely linked with their interest in and empathy for older people was the positive reaction which some helpers described on hearing about the scheme. They may not have been looking for this kind of work but the scheme sounded such a good idea that they wanted to participate. Helpers were asked specifically what kind of things they were considering doing at the time they applied to the scheme. Over one-third stated that they had not intended to do anything else but were stimulated by hearing about the scheme. One helper described herself as having been 'grabbed' by the advertisement in the paper. Their own experiences of caring had taught them how much help older people might need, and they were enthusiastic about more help being offered. In particular, they were keen to help older people remain in their own homes. One helper sensed an immediate match between herself and the scheme's objectives because of personal experiences:

> It [the application] was done on the spur of the moment really. The scheme sounded interesting and I was thinking of getting some kind of part-time work. My mother had dementia and was in hospital for two years. I felt, after that, as if I'd like to keep other people out of hospital.

Similar personal experiences motivated some of her colleagues, as did some people's work experiences. Helpers who had worked in care homes or long-stay geriatric wards were sometimes almost evangelistic in their desire to save older people from institutionalisation. Other helpers talked of the loneliness and isolation of frail older people who had no family care network, and felt that a scheme that would fill this care gap was worthy of their support.

*Social giving* It has been seen that helpers saw the scheme as offering them a range of material and psychological rewards. It often appealed to their sense of what was right for older people. Intermingled with these themes, however, was a sense of altruism or generalised reciprocity (Bulmer, 1986; Qureshi et al., 1989); a desire to give to others for its own sake, or to make their contribution to the overall pool of social giving from which they also needed to receive. Unlike Titmuss's (1970) blood donor sample, the helpers were not explicitly asked to give without return, or to donate their care anonymously. Equally, a substantial number did not attach much initial importance to financial reward, and when helpers offered their services, it was not usually with a particular individual in mind. They were offering their help to an unspecified stranger (see item 2 in Table 4.4) and undertaking socially valued activity (see item 1). Many helpers included in their overall comments on their motivation, general indications such as 'I just like to help people'.

Their altruistic inclinations were illustrated by the voluntary caring many were doing in their neighbourhoods both before and while they worked for the scheme. Some said they had not realised that they would receive payment when they joined the scheme. Others made it clear that although a financial element was important, it did not detract from their desire to give of themselves to needy people in the community:

I would do it voluntary if I wasn't paid, but the bit of independence is very nice. It's an emotional job; you have to want to do it. You wouldn't just do it for the money.

Sometimes past personal experiences had made helpers especially sensitive to the need for people to help each other:

I particularly wanted to help an old person who didn't have any family of their own and who was lonely. I was lonely as a child. I think that's what makes me want to help a lonely old person.

Others anticipated reciprocal help in the future:

I was asked (by another helper) if I was interested in helping old people. I thought it was a good scheme, and something I ought to do, because I'll be old one day, and would like to think there'd be something like that for me.

These sentiments are evidenced by item 12 in Table 4.4. Item 10 indicates that almost one-third of helpers felt it was a moral or religious imperative to help others, and this is illustrated by some of their comments:

I think everybody ought to help people, but some people just aren't suitable.

This view of helping was significantly greater in the outer city area. These helpers seemed to have a strong sense of what Titmuss called 'building the fabric of social values' (Titmuss, 1970). Looking after an old person now neither undid past sadness nor guaranteed help if it was needed in the future. Helping people was not rewarded by direct offers of reciprocal help; but it made a statement about the desirability of establishing certain kinds of values and human support networks which would be of general social benefit, and some helpers certainly wanted to contribute to this.

*Common elements in motivational themes* It has been seen that helpers' motivations were multiple and the themes elaborated here are based on the answers which helpers themselves gave to specific questions about their motivation. There is no doubt from the data that the more expressive aspect of the scheme was a major attraction and often singled out this work from other kinds of comparable employment available to these people. Nevertheless, it would be wrong to allow this to obscure the importance of more material considerations.

Even those helpers for whom money was not an essential element found the extra cash very useful both in terms of what it could buy and in terms of the personal autonomy and increased self respect which their own earnings could buy. Similarly, the practical accessibility of the scheme as an activity was very influential. It offered work at times and in forms which women could take, whilst retaining their primary commitment to their families. Moreover, it enabled women to take time out of their family obligations, without causing any unmanageable disruption to their pattern of life. It offered an outlet outside the home without in any way challenging their role within it. Indeed, it could be seen as an extension of that role, but with the added interest of being part of an organised scheme, and meeting new people outside their own families.

Others have discussed that it is not sufficient to explain volunteers' motivation by reference to their 'concern for others', as many people who do not volunteer may also display such concern (Hadley et al., 1975; Leat, 1983). The Gateshead helpers would score highly on a measure of 'concern for others', but the attraction for them was the fact that the scheme not only gave them an opportunity to express their caring qualities, but was also a practical proposition in terms of finance, location and what they could offer to do in their specific social context. Thus latent motivations can only become manifest when the context permits. The next two sections consider the helpers' context more fully, by examining the factors associated with different types of motivation and the extent to which different types of motivation occurred together in helpers.

### Specific motivations and factors associated with their presence

In the preceding section the broad themes that emerged from helpers' discussions of aspects of motivation were considered. Here an examination is made of the extent to which helpers' personal characteristics and situations were associated with particular motivations.

The importance of the nature and extent of motivation in helpers is clear. This information will have a bearing on both the types of work that a particular helper will prefer and their degree of commitment. In order to gain some insight into how different helpers tend to be motivated in varying ways which relate to what they were willing to do, it is useful to examine to what extent different types of motivation are associated with different individual characteristics. This has been undertaken by means of a logistic regression analysis for each type of motivation, using characteristics of the helper and the number of types of different tasks that the helpers performed as predictors.

Unsurprisingly, the success with which different types of motivation could be predicted varied widely. It was decided to restrict further consideration to those motivations where there was a reasonable prediction of the probability of having a particular motivation. These are now considered in turn. Thus, only those motivations where more than 35 per cent of the variation in the presence/absence of the motivation could be explained are considered, and the findings discussed in summary form.

*An interest outside the home or separate identity* This group of helpers were more likely to be located in the outer city, and were generally much younger than helpers as a whole. They were unlikely to have been in employment at the time of selection. A number had previous caring experience as a nursing auxiliary or home help, but they were unlikely to have had social services experience in a residential home or day centre. Some of the group had low levels of income as a result mainly of unemployment in the family. This resulted in their receiving state benefit, which sometimes led to problems with the benefit or tax authorities.

*To look after or care for someone (altruism-personality)* These helpers tended to be slightly younger and have fewer children at home. Fewer were owner-occupiers. Fewer were recruited through the older person or through a voluntary organisation, and fewer had voluntary experience. Problems with the benefit or tax authorities were also less frequent. There were fewer helpers in the professional/technical, white collar and unskilled socio-economic groups. As expected, a greater range of household and personal care tasks was performed but fewer tasks related to social and emotional needs or contact with others involved.

*To work with the elderly (altruism-empathy)* Those wishing to work with older people tended to be a little younger and were unlikely to have children at home. They were not normally recruited through the older person's informal network or through another helper. Recruitment through advertising did not feature highly. These helpers more frequently had training as a nurse or nursing auxiliary, though helpers with voluntary experience were less likely to be represented. The socio-economic groups of professional/technical, white collar and unskilled manual were less likely to be motivated by work with older people. Helpers were more likely to perform a wider range of personal care tasks but were less likely to take part in tasks directed towards social or emotional needs, or in liaising with many parts of the caring network.

*To help someone in need* These helpers were more likely to be located in the outer city and were on average slightly older. They were less likely to be widowed, separated or divorced. The proportion who were owner-occupiers was less and fewer were from families of 'white collar' status.

These helpers were involved in a smaller range of tasks that tackled social or emotional needs, or involving liaison with the caring network.

*Something anyone in my position ought to do, social obligation (reciprocity)* Helpers in the outer city were more likely to be included in this group, together with people who were normally employed in a caring occupation or as a housewife. However, they were less likely to have children at home. Mothers whose children had grown up and left home had a greater feeling of social obligation. A slightly greater proportion was recruited through the older person and slightly fewer through advertising. Rather more were in employment at the time of recruitment, though more had voluntary experience. More of the group were of professional/technical socio-economic status. These helpers had contact with a wider range of the caring network.

*To take my mind off my own worries (diversion or therapy)* These helpers were more likely to be located in the outer city and to be owner-occupiers. They were more frequently recruited through the older person or their informal network or other helpers. Helpers with previous experience as home helps were more likely to be in this category. Their socio-economic status tended to be skilled or unskilled manual. It was found that the group did not take part in as wide a range of personal care tasks and did not maintain as much contact with other parties involved in the care, but performed a wider variety of tasks related to social or emotional needs.

*To use my skills/knowledge* This group of helpers tended to be somewhat older. As expected, many more had experience in caring, and rather more were in employment at the time of recruitment. Fewer were recruited through other helpers. They were much more likely to have previous experience in residential homes, day centres or voluntary work. Rather more were from the skilled and also unemployed socio-economic groups. It was found that this group were more likely to perform a wide range of personal care tasks.

Thus, different motivations appeared to be experienced by individuals in different circumstances, although distinction cannot be too clear-cut given the multiplicity of motives held by individuals.

### The clustering of motivations

In practice individuals expressed several motivations concurrently. To what extent were there consistent patterns? The relative importance of fourteen different possible motivations for helpers joining the scheme has already been described in Table 4.4. A cluster analysis (Romesburg, 1984) by helper based upon these fourteen indicators suggested that helpers fell naturally into eight clusters. As three of these clusters consisted of only one helper and another of only two, these were excluded, leaving four main groups. The distinguishing features of each group are now briefly described.

*Group 1 — personal altruism* This was by far the largest group, accounting for some two-thirds of all helpers. This group were mostly *not* motivated by the wish to fill their spare time or be stimulated, though over half wanted to earn some money. They did not on the whole want to repay help received. All but one wished to look after someone (personal altruism). The few helpers wanting to take their mind off their own worries (diversion) were mainly included in this group. Nearly half wished to use their skills or knowledge.

*Group 2 — payment* This group of fifteen helpers had a fairly high proportion (60 per cent) located in the inner city, compared with only 38 per cent for helpers as a whole, which reflected their economic circumstances. Some two-thirds of them specifically wished to earn some money. Reflecting this greater focus on instrumental factors, none of them wanted to help someone in need, and only one-third of the group wished to meet people. Few wanted to repay help received. Only 13 per cent wished to look after someone, and a similar proportion wanted to use their skills or knowledge. Very few saw the work as offering experience for a job or career. None of the group saw the work as meeting a social obligation. Regarding the rewards obtained, none of them experienced an improved social life, and only one helper in five found greater personal independence. Nevertheless, there was little evidence of a wish to leave the scheme, the main reasons for leaving being too much pressure or a change in personal or family circumstances.

*Group 3 — Independence/human capital building/time to spare/useful/affiliation* This group of seventeen helpers were all seeking an interest outside the home (independence), and nearly half wanted experience for a job or career (human capital building). Seventy-one per cent wished to repay help received (reciprocity). This group is therefore similar to the independence/human capital building cluster of Qureshi et al. (1989) for helpers in Kent. Most of the group were located in the outer city and very few had previous voluntary experience. Nearly all wished to meet people (affiliation) and all of them wanted to work with older people and to help someone in need. Over three-quarters wished to fill their spare time or derive stimulation and 94 per cent saw it as a chance to be useful. The group, therefore, also bears similarity with the 'time to spare/useful/affiliation' cluster of Qureshi et al. (1989). Only one helper in four wished to earn money. Thus the independence sought was on the whole not financial. In fact, some two-thirds saw the work as a social obligation (reciprocity).

Regarding the rewards derived for this group, all helpers felt a respect or attachment to the older person, and nearly all obtained a sense of their own achievement. Seventy-one per cent found it kept them occupied, and over half had obtained career experience (human capital building). Forty-one per cent had an improved social life, and two-thirds obtained greater personal independence.

A number of these helpers had left or considered leaving the scheme. The main reason for leaving was alternative employment (29 per cent) which is a natural consequence for the human capital building element in the group. Also 18 per cent complained of insufficient work, and a similar proportion of insufficient pay. However, none of them complained of too much pressure arising from their participation in the scheme.

*Group 4 — personal altruism/reciprocity* This small group of only four helpers were located entirely in the outer city. None of them joined the scheme with a definite wish to earn some money. None of them had been explicitly seeking work with older people, though all wanted to help someone in need and to look after someone (personal altruism). All of them wished to repay help received (reciprocity). Although none saw the work as experience for a job or career, half of them welcomed the opportunity to use their skills or knowledge. Three-quarters saw the work as honouring a social obligation (reciprocity).

The entire group was rewarded by the older person's gratitude or appreciation and by being needed. However, only one helper enjoyed a feeling of responsibility as a reward for the work. None found it improved their social life and only one found it had developed their own education or skills. However, three-quarters found it gave them greater personal independence.

Thus helpers with different clusters of motivations tended to be in different circumstances. The next section examines their experiences of providing help.


## Working with older people

Although one half of the helpers interviewed started work within one month of being accepted, 11 per cent had to wait for over six months, reflecting the difficulties in successful matching between helpers and older people. However, this was only rarely seen to be a real problem for the helper. Delay was more frequent for helpers from the outer city, probably due to their greater geographical dispersion. Training was provided for a substantial number of helpers and the content of this was discussed in the previous chapter.

Although the older person was already well known to the helper before joining the scheme in only a few cases, 46 per cent of helpers were still visiting their first older person when interviewed, indicating how time permitted close relationships to develop. Over half of the helpers (55 per cent) found the experience of the scheme coincided largely with their expectations, a few finding it much better and a few much worse.

At the time the helpers were interviewed 71 per cent were currently working for the scheme. Of these, well over half were visiting older people on at least five days per week and over a quarter were visiting daily. Over three-quarters worked for over five hours per week, and nearly half worked for ten hours weekly. Seventy per cent of helpers worked more or less continuously for the scheme even if they eventually withdrew. The main reason for gaps in the work was due to none being available from the scheme, which was a greater problem in the outer city where geographical matching between helper and older person was harder to achieve. This lack of regular, guaranteed employment, caused some difficulty to nearly a quarter of helpers. Overall, it is noteworthy that more than half the helpers (58 per cent) would have preferred to be a regular employee, with regular hours, although with considerably greater flexibility than usually exists in home care work.

### Tasks undertaken

What then were the tasks undertaken by helpers and to what extent did different helpers tend to undertake different tasks? Information on helper tasks was based on a survey of 68 helpers over a four-week period, providing a total of 272 helper weeks. The range of tasks undertaken by helpers was very wide, as can be seen from Tables 4.5, 4.6 and 4.7. A considerable amount of activity was undertaken ensuring adequate diet, providing personal care, helping to manage incontinence, giving social support, and assisting people with dementia through reassurance and reality orientation. Other therapeutic activities were undertaken by helpers less frequently, such as helping older people to re-acquire skills such as dressing, or working under the supervision of a physiotherapist following a stroke to improve mobility. Tasks not noted here included activities which helpers undertook beyond what was specified in their contract, such as taking people on outings. Table 4.5 shows the wide extent of household tasks that were undertaken, ranging from shopping to sewing. The most frequently performed activities were concerned with meal preparation. These took a variety of different forms, including helpers preparing meals in their own homes. Occasionally, other activities such as pet care, important to the older people but often not readily undertaken by services, were also undertaken.

With regard to personal care, Table 4.6 indicates that the main activities were associated with rising and retiring, including dressing and grooming. The range of activities extended from assistance with activities of daily living, such as toileting and transfer, to the management of medication and more specifically nursing tasks. In a few cases both night and day sitting were tasks undertaken.

Table 4.7 shows the range of support tasks which helpers undertook. These ranged from general companionship to more identifiably therapeutic activities, such as reality orientation. Some of the activities were specifically rehabilitative, encouraging people to re-acquire skills that had become impaired. These activities ranged well beyond what would have been expected of any

**Table 4.5**
*The frequency with which household tasks were undertaken[a]*

| Task | | Helper weeks % |
|---|---|---|
| Housework: | clean or tidy | 58 |
| | make or change bed | 56 |
| Errands: | regular shopping | 52 |
| | occasional shopping e.g. clothing | 7 |
| | collect prescription or pension | 29 |
| Laundry: | heavy laundry | 6 |
| | wash soiled items | 22 |
| | personal/light laundry | 40 |
| Meals: | prepare meal, drink or snack in older person's home | 91 |
| | take meal from helper's home | 34 |
| | throw away stale food | 50 |
| | keep a check on the amount older person has eaten or drunk | 22 |
| | wash up | 89 |
| | supervise meals-on-wheels | 12 |
| Heating: | light or maintain fire or fetch coal | 32 |
| | help with heating system e.g. gas or electric fires or central heating | 34 |
| Other tasks: | odd jobs e.g. mend items, change plugs, home maintenance | 12 |
| | regular small tasks e.g. wind clocks, change calendar, put clothes out or away | 68 |
| | sewing | 11 |
| | help find mislaid or removed items | 29 |
| | see to cigarettes or pipe | 9 |
| | pet care: e.g. exercise, clean up, feed | 8 |
| | hold older person's door key | 49 |
| Finances: | pay bills or rent | 14 |
| | assist in household finances and business | 18 |

a  Sample size: 272 helper weeks from 68 helpers.

home care service. Aspects of service development were also noted, such as running a day group in helpers' own homes.

For ease of analysis, these tasks were grouped together in eleven areas: weekly household tasks; daily household tasks; help with meals; making snacks and drinks; rising and retiring; daily and weekly personal care; help to carers; companionship; emotional support; rehabilitation and reality orientation; assessment/understanding older person's needs. In order to examine whether or not there were patterns in the type of activities that were undertaken a cluster analysis was performed, using the eleven task areas listed above. Six clusters of helper task groups were identified, although most of these groups represented but a few helpers. Unsurprisingly, it appeared that

**Table 4.6**
*The frequency with which personal care tasks were undertaken*[a]

| Task | | Helper weeks % |
|---|---|---|
| Bed-time: | personal care tasks involved with getting up or putting to bed | 71 |
| | lock or unlock house | 59 |
| Dressing: | help with dressing or undressing | 64 |
| | change soiled clothes | 37 |
| Other care: | groom hair or shave | 62 |
| | cut or clean toenails | 6 |
| | cut or clean fingernails | 15 |
| Toileting: | help with toilet or onto commode | 41 |
| | clean or empty commode, bottle or bed pan | 57 |
| | change or dispose of incontinence pads or sheets | 21 |
| | clean up faeces, urine, vomit, sputum | 18 |
| Medication: | give or check tablets or medicine | 66 |
| | order prescription direct from surgery | 11 |
| | apply drops, cream or ointment/change dressing or bandages | 28 |
| Bath or wash | | 51 |
| Night sitting for all or part of night | | 5 |
| Appointments, e.g. accompany to doctor, hospital, chiropodist etc. | | 4 |
| Respond to emergency, e.g. after fall or sudden illness | | 4 |
| Day sitting to relieve family or other carer | | 7 |
| Appliances: | help with false limbs or other aids e.g. calliper | 6 |
| | attend to hearing aid, false teeth, spectacles | 31 |
| Special nursing task, e.g. attend to pressure sores | | 3 |

a  Sample size: 272 helper weeks from 68 helpers.

most helpers were relatively generic in the range of activities they undertook, although a few focused upon a more limited range involving companionship, assessment, assisting carers, rehabilitation and reality orientation. Those who undertook this latter range of more specialised and, at times, therapeutic tasks, were less likely to also undertake the full range of household and personal care.

These analyses suggest that most helpers undertook most caring tasks. However, there were small numbers who undertook less personal care, or gave help only at specific times, or who undertook sitting and other supportive activities. Clearly, finding the helpers to undertake the right 'mix' of activities at the right time for a particular person was critical.

**Table 4.7**
*The frequency with which support tasks were undertaken*[a]

| Task | Helper weeks % |
|---|---|
| *Companionship and stimulation:* | |
| sit and chat, stimulate interest | 88 |
| help with handicrafts or leisure activities | 11 |
| *Rehabilitation/encouraging independence:* | |
| exercises, improve mobility | 8 |
| teach or encourage older person to learn to toilet self | 8 |
| teach or encourage older person to learn to dress self | 10 |
| teach or encourage older person to learn to wash self | 8 |
| take for shopping/outings and help join social activities outside home | 18 |
| help older person to prepare meal | 3 |
| help older person with behaviour, attitude, relationships | 15 |
| *Reality orientation:* | |
| remind older person regarding time, place or person | 39 |
| tidy up after confused older person | 16 |
| provide reassurance or calm | 25 |
| Provide transport | 10 |
| Assist with running a day group | 7 |
| Deal with telephone calls or correspondence | 23 |
| Visit older person in hospital, residential care etc. | 3 |

a   Sample size: 272 helper weeks from 68 helpers.

## Relationship with older person

Bearing in mind that many older people are used to leading an independent life and might be reluctant to accept help from strangers, the vast majority of helpers experienced older people as being highly appreciative and only 8 per cent of helpers reported them as being consistently difficult to please. Only a very few helpers felt that being paid made it more difficult for people to accept their help, and in fact one in four thought that payment made it easier for help to be accepted. Moreover, about 40 per cent of helpers felt that working as part of an official social services scheme made it easier for the older person. Some four helpers in every five felt that people were better off at home and felt a strong commitment to their continued independence. Where a concern about living at home was expressed, about 6 per cent favoured sheltered housing, a further 6 per cent residential care and 2 per cent hospital. Helpers' families also frequently became involved in visiting the older person, and in fact, only 28 per cent never visited. Indeed, in about 10 per cent of cases the older person was visiting the helper's home at least monthly.

*Relationship with informal carers*

Although relatively few carers were seen on a more or less daily basis, about one helper in three saw a family member at least once a week, and found their contact very helpful for moral support, sharing of responsibility or information. Although one in five helpers experienced some difficulties with the older person's family, in very few cases were these were substantial. Usually, such problems were only minor, and the helper was able to overcome them.

One principle of the scheme was not to undermine existing informal support. Rather, it aimed to build around the informal support already present and some 85 per cent of helpers had developed friendships with the older person's family. About one half of helpers reported no consequent change upon the level of family help and only one found an increase in help. However, about a quarter found the family did less, perhaps reflecting the provision of a degree of relief.

Over half (60 per cent) of helpers knew of friends or neighbours that helped the older person, and about one-third of helpers had at least weekly contact with them. Although a far smaller proportion of helpers shared tasks with them than with the family, the contact was again experienced as important for moral support or sharing of responsibility or information. Interestingly, helpers identified fewer difficulties with friends and neighbours than they did with the older person's family, and experienced little hindrance, perhaps because the pressures and ambivalence of these supporters were much less. For those older people with friends or neighbours who helped, the involvement of the scheme had less effect in reducing the informal support given than it did with the family, only 12 per cent reporting a reduction in support.

*Supervision and support*

As part of the specification of their role, helpers received a contract from the scheme explaining whom they helped, what they were to do and what they were trying to achieve. The contract given to a helper would spell out the essential tasks and visits required for each person. One aspect of flexibility was to permit helpers to feel free to build upon this basic involvement and use their initiative to respond more effectively to the older person's needs. Although about one helper in every four usually stuck to the contract, most used the contract simply as providing broad guidelines, particularly when they felt that their own perception of needs was not sufficiently catered for in the contract. Consequently, nearly one half of helpers (46 per cent) regularly made extra visits or performed additional tasks not specified in the contract.

Contact between care manager and helper, either face-to-face or by telephone, was relatively frequent. Most helpers were split evenly between those having contact with the care manager at least once a week (27 per cent), fortnightly (28 per cent) and monthly (29 per cent). This contact was more often initiated by the care manager, and did not show much change over time for most helpers, though any change was towards less contact as the helper became more experienced. The vast majority found the contact both useful and sufficient. The reasons for contact between care managers and helpers are shown in Table 4.8. As expected, most saw contact as concerned with general monitoring, and three-quarters were in contact over relief cover. Two-thirds were in contact over sudden changes in the older person's state, identifying the need for reassessment and extra intervention. Other factors necessitating contact were sudden changes in the support network and relationship/coordination difficulties with other carers. More than half of the helpers were sometimes advised by the care manager as to how to cope with the older person. Support was provided when mediation with other agencies or informal carers was required. Indeed, nearly half the helpers were in touch with the care manager for emotional or moral support. Finally, nearly half had been in touch regarding the administration of their payment. Only one helper in seven sometimes experienced difficulty in contacting the care manager when needed. Very few helpers reported disagreement with the care managers' decisions.

**Table 4.8**
*Type of contact between helper and care manager*

| Type of contact | % |
| --- | --- |
| General monitoring/keeping in touch about older person | 92 |
| Need for relief cover | 77 |
| Sudden change in older person's state | 66 |
| Mediation with agencies/carers | 61 |
| Advice on tasks/role of helper | 57 |
| Emotional/moral support for helper | 48 |
| Personal administrative problems (pay, tax etc.) | 45 |
| Relationship difficulties with older person | 35 |
| Relationship/coordination difficulties with other carers | 26 |
| Sudden change in support network | 13 |
| Assessment/reassessment of older person's need (at care manager's request) | 3 |
| Number of helpers = 119 | |

Half of the helpers normally used their own judgement in dealing with situations, needing minimal guidance or support from the care manager. A further third required a moderate degree of advice from the care manager but still relied substantially on their own judgement. As experience grew, so did the degree of self-reliance reported by helpers.

Helpers met each other frequently. The main type of contact with other helpers was through sharing responsibilities or activities or through regular relief work (68 per cent). A further 15 per cent met other helpers informally through their own network. Helpers benefited from this contact in a number of ways. Three-quarters of helpers found it helped with specific activities, and two-thirds found it provided general support or guidance. Meeting other helpers had the additional benefit of improving their social life. Although nearly half of the helpers (46 per cent) found this contact sufficient, or indeed preferred to work alone, one-third would have liked more general mutual support or contact. This suggested the need for a wider range of group activity such as the training courses, which proved useful for most helpers who had received them.

## Contact with other agencies

Overall, contact between helpers and other agencies was nearly all experienced as helpful. One-third of all helpers had regular helpful contact with the home help, 15 per cent with the community nurse and a similar proportion with the housing warden. Contact with the general practitioner, although mostly helpful, was less frequent. The only areas where contact was seen as not particularly helpful were with housing wardens and general practitioners, but only in a few cases. This arose due to the perspective of both parties that enhanced community care may significantly increase their workload. To the housing warden it was the demands of a vulnerable older person whose needs and demands were greater than most residents. For some general practitioners the extra demands on their time led to their refusing to be called out by the helper at times of illness, particularly during out of office hours when the helper had least access to other forms of help.

## Multiplier effects

As part of an overall evaluation of the benefits of the scheme, it is interesting to consider the extent to which the involvement of helpers proved catalytic in influencing them to extend their helping role to people outside the scheme. This reflects the concept of a 'reciprocity multiplier' (Gouldner, 1960; Qureshi et al., 1989). One helper in four had also become involved in helping someone outside the scheme, particularly a neighbour or a relative. However, in only a minority of these cases was the involvement prompted by work for the scheme. Similarly, 8 per cent of helpers had given up helping someone whom they used to assist before working for the scheme. Thus, although on balance 16 per cent more helpers were assisting people outside the scheme, only a quarter of this change was attributed to the scheme. There was no apparent effect upon their involvement in organised voluntary activity.

**Bridging formal and informal care: the helper role**

Despite the perceived advantages of being a paid helper working for an agency, nearly half the helpers saw themselves as much as a friend of the older person or part of the family, and a further one-third of helpers found the work more than a job, although they did not see themselves in the role of a friend. Very few helpers saw it as mainly a job. Responding to a hypothetical question of the scheme being discontinued after the trial period, 8 per cent of helpers felt they would continue to maintain the same level of contact with the older person, and 49 per cent thought they would continue to visit but at a lower level of contact. A further 14 per cent of helpers felt they would continue to visit some of the older people. Thus very few of the helpers still in the scheme felt they would cease contact altogether.

Equally, earning money was seen as important for nearly two-thirds of helpers although not necessarily a prime motive. Over half the helpers felt that the pay they received was about right for the work required or very good. Only 4 per cent of helpers were very dissatisfied, and a similar proportion had approached the care manager about a pay increase, about half of whom had been successful. A few more had not felt able to raise the subject. However, it is noteworthy that the vast majority (82 per cent) never felt the need to ask for a pay increase. Nonetheless, nearly all helpers preferred being paid. Only one helper felt it better to be unpaid.

Two obvious policy questions arise regarding the status of helpers and their payment. Firstly, what are the respective roles of paid and volunteer carers in the provision of this kind of community support for very dependent people. On the one hand, is it necessary to pay people in order to secure good neighbourhood care? On the other hand, is it feasible or ethical not to do so? Secondly, what lies behind the caring motivation expressed by the helpers and what implication does this have for their role in organised community care?

*Employee or volunteer*

There are clear conflicts between a model of organised care for the very frail and the expression of a caring society and the 'natural' duty of family networks and local communities. There is a fear of a 'commercialisation effect', that paying people to provide care eventually backfires by discouraging people from offering the help they would otherwise give freely (Hirsch, 1977; Land, 1978). At a policy level, one interpretation of the focus upon support of carers reflects a need to achieve a new balance between payment and obligation. It is useful to explore the helpers' responses to the issue of payment in more detail.

Almost all of them regarded the payments they received as an integral and essential part of their contract with the scheme. As has been seen, many of them needed money to the point that they could not otherwise have worked for the scheme, but their attitude to being paid was much more complex than that. Some did not feel a pressing need to earn money and said that they would have joined the scheme even if no payment had been offered. Nonetheless, payment was only refused by a very small number of helpers who were barred by their receipt of certain state benefits from earning anything at all. Virtually all helpers were clear that the job should be paid rather than unpaid. A variety of reasons other than financial need were described. One was the formal recognition and acknowledgement which payment bestowed on the service which helpers were providing. It was a symbol that their contribution was valuable and appreciated even if it did not fully equate with the effort that they put in. Secondly, helpers felt that being paid by a statutory body gave them the status they needed in the eyes of the older people and their families. It meant that they could insist confidently on doing their job, even in difficult circumstances, because it had the paid status of employment.

One helper illustrated the sort of resistance she would anticipate if she was a volunteer. She felt that if she was not paid and official her motives would be under suspicion: 'They'd think you were after something'.

Another helper had different worries:

Helpers should be paid — it makes it easier for the old people and their families to accept help, and not feel it's charity. Families feel that it is easier to ask helpers to change their hours or do extra, if they know they are being paid, and not giving the time voluntarily.

Other helpers experienced conflicts with the older person's family or with employees of other services, and felt that they would have been disadvantaged if they had no official paid status.

A third reason given was that helpers' own commitment might be diminished if the contract was not sealed by some kind of payment. As one helper said: 'They (paid workers) are more reliable and dependable than if they were volunteers'.

Another said that without pay:

Helpers wouldn't do as much so regularly. They might visit occasionally but not to do the same things. You wouldn't commit yourself.

Some helpers made explicit distinctions between the sort of work which fell legitimately into the voluntary sphere and that which did not. Bringing it right down to basics, one helper said:

You do more (if you are paid). I wouldn't have emptied the commode if I'd not been paid; I'd have left it for the home help to do it as it was her job and she was getting paid.

Another helper said:

I wouldn't mind doing voluntary work in hospitals — visiting people and taking the trolleys round and that kind of thing, but for the sort of work we do (for the scheme), I think you should get paid.

On a more personal note, helpers deeply appreciated the additional independence their earnings gave them. Even those who did not anticipate initially that this would be important, soon realised how much it meant to them:

> I enjoy the job; the money is less important..., but it is better to be paid. I like getting the money and it's nice to feel I'm earning something...., I like to have a bit of money for myself, whether I spend it on the house or not.

Thus, helpers felt they should be paid; were motivated to do more caring, not less, because they were receiving money for doing it; and it appeared unlikely that they would have felt able or willing to fulfil the helper's role as comprehensively and continuously, if they had been expected to do it for nothing. As with Kent helpers, payment was a necessary but rarely a sufficient condition for participation. This is consistent with Abram's finding in the Stonegate Warden Scheme: '...far from being incompatible with paid work, a distinctively working class pattern of care was in fact dependent on it and could flourish on the basis of it' (Bulmer, 1986, p.212).

### An opportunity or exploitation?

The most striking characteristic of the helpers in the Gateshead and Kent schemes was that they were usually female. They had this in common with all the other reported schemes seeking to provide intensive support to dependent groups. As Finch (1984) points out, such schemes tend to involve 'creating new categories of low paid workers who undertake and organise daily caring', and 'they often build upon an extension of domestic virtues believed to be the especial property of women. Moreover, the 'caring' envisaged in such schemes implies not just domestic work but a qualitative relationship with the dependent person, of a type characteristically assigned to women in our culture' (p10). It has been seen that Gateshead helpers were attracted to the scheme precisely because it offered them accessible paid work, which offered an opportunity for them to use the skills and experience which being a primary carer in the family had given them, and which gave expression to the sort of caring identity which they had adopted for themselves and which clearly fits in with cultural expectations of what women should be. Yet aspects which subjectively may be a source of attraction for helpers, may be also simultaneously a potential source of their exploitation. While women are seen as society's 'natural' unpaid carers, and while they see themselves as responsible for giving freely of themselves for this purpose, their bargaining power in the labour market will be weak. The helpers in Gateshead had a primary commitment to their unpaid work as wives and mothers, and their employment opportunities were therefore limited to work which would not detract from these commitments. As Hilary Land (1978) argues, beliefs which accord women the main responsibility for caring for other family members, ensure a constant supply of women who are prepared to offer their labour on terms which are favourable to employers. It could be argued that the helpers were doing exactly this. The work they were being offered was relatively low paid and had a casual status. It carried none of the rights and benefits of a conventional job, such as guaranteed hours or income. Helpers sacrificed such benefits in order to get a job which did not specify hours of work which they found difficult to reconcile with their families, but which at least produced some income, however modest, and which yielded more job satisfaction than conventional female manual employment.

Furthermore, the association of this kind of work with the caring identity culturally attributed to women laid the helpers open not only to an exploitation of their material circumstances, but also of their goodwill. They displayed a keen awareness of the needs and rights of the older people, mainly other women, whom they were offering to help. Many often acknowledged the needs of the supporting relatives, usually also other women, for relief. They recognised the value of a scheme which sought to improve the quality of life of such needy people, and were very unhappy at the thought of them being neglected, or admitted reluctantly to institutions. Their emotional response to the need for care, and the moral imperative felt by women to offer care when care is needed, made it difficult for them to give their own needs and rights a high profile.

Viewed thus, the scheme did not offer what Finch (1984) would describe as 'non-sexist community care', any more than do other caring services. Like these, it relied on women's view of themselves as carers, and women's availability to perform modestly paid work at hours convenient to their employers. Nevertheless, it is important to balance this against the much more positive subjective experience of the helpers. Within the socio-economic context in which they lived, the scheme offered a much more satisfying and convenient work setting than most others available to them, and this is why they were so highly motivated to join it. Alternative employment open to them did not necessarily offer better conditions, and even if it did, it typically failed to offer equivalent personal satisfaction. As such the scheme constituted an additional 'opportunity' (Evers, 1994).

The helpers interviewed wanted to feel that they would be achieving something worthwhile and useful and which would bring emotional rewards as well as material ones. They saw the scheme as an opportunity to develop aspects of themselves which they valued, whilst not having to neglect their family identities, which they also valued. Their part in the scheme, certainly, did not challenge the role of women as society's carers, but it at least seemed to offer a more independent and rewarding context in which women could practice their skills and receive recognition for them. Leat and Gay (1987) have suggested that this balancing of objectives by the helpers reflects a 'rationality of care' which renders paid care schemes less exploitative than other forms of care giving. 'Within the rationality of caring, payment and care are not antithetical — payment does not negate caring just as non-payment does not guarantee it. Equally, however, payment does not have the same significance as in other types of work and systems of rationality in which calculations of cost and benefit are primary' (p.62).

Overall the analysis suggests that the provision of payment and of working conditions which are not too disruptive of family life were major factors in attracting local women with families to offer their services as helpers, but it is important also not to lose sight of the job satisfaction and emotional rewards which helpers hoped to get from this kind of work. Both aspects together added up to a highly motivated workforce. There are, however, dangers which must be guarded against, in particular the vulnerability of such workforce to exploitation; and this places a particular responsibility on the organisers of such schemes (Leat and Gay, 1987; Qureshi et al., 1983, 1989; Ungerson, 1993). They cannot offer a solution to issues of social disadvantage (Baldock and Ungerson, 1991) but they can at least address themselves to questions of rights and safeguards for their workforce on the job. If they do not, they risk not only allegations of exploitation, but also of losing the 'best' helpers who, if their motivations do not find fulfilment, will seek alternative outlets. Payment for care raises moral and political issues along with the more immediate gains (Ungerson, 1994).

## Satisfaction and drawbacks of being a helper

Since continuity and stability in patterns of care are likely to be indicative of quality, it is helpful to understand the factors that encouraged and discouraged them in their work.

Helpers were asked about a number of possible rewards that they might have derived from the work. The responses are shown in Table 4.9. Six rewards were found by nearly all helpers: a sense of purpose/worthwhile activity (97 per cent); an improvement in the person's welfare or quality of life (86 per cent); respect for/emotional attachment to the older person (86 per cent); feelings of indispensability or being needed (84 per cent); sense of own achievement in successful caring (82 per cent); and appreciation/gratitude of the older person (80 per cent).

Over half of the helpers (58 per cent) enjoyed taking on responsibility and about half found the work useful to fill time. The work was useful in providing career experience or professional contact for 40 per cent of helpers. A feeling of greater personal independence was expressed by 37 per cent of helpers. About one helper in three reported a development of their own education or skills. Finally the work improved social life or allowed the helper to meet others in 18 per cent of cases.

Helpers were also asked whether they experienced any of a range of possible difficulties in their role. The responses are shown in Table 4.10. Thirty-nine per cent had at some stage encountered difficulties in the personality and attitudes of an older person. In view of the extensiveness of ill health, including

**Table 4.9**
*Rewards of the scheme for the helpers*

| Reward | % |
| --- | --- |
| Sense of purpose/worthwhile activity | 97 |
| Improvement in older person's welfare/quality of life | 86 |
| Respect for/emotional attachment to older person | 86 |
| Feeling indispensable/needed by older person | 84 |
| Sense of own achievement in successful caring | 82 |
| Appreciation/gratitude of older person | 80 |
| Enjoyment of taking responsibility | 58 |
| Something to do/filling in time | 49 |
| Career experience/professional contact | 40 |
| Greater personal independence | 37 |
| Development of own education/skills | 35 |
| Improved social life/meeting others | 18 |

Number of helpers = 119

dementia and other difficulties, this figure is perhaps at a level to be expected. A quarter of helpers found the nature of the illness or the extent of frailty a problem at times, often reflecting their felt difficulty at leaving people knowing that no one else may be available to visit for some time. One helper in five found confusion a difficulty, which is perhaps hardly surprising and 13 per cent of helpers found the deafness, poor speech or communication difficulties a problem. One helper in five found reluctance to accept help a problem, and slightly fewer encountered problems with other agencies. Other difficulties arose over disputes over money management with the older person or carer and dirty, impoverished and ill-equipped homes.

For about a quarter of the helpers an obligation to do things that they would have preferred not to do had been experienced. The tasks most frequently mentioned were dressing and undressing (9 per cent), getting up and putting to bed (6 per cent), bathing or washing down (4 per cent) and toileting/commode emptying (4 per cent). The pressure to perform these unwelcome tasks came mainly from the helper's own assessment of need and their feeling of worry or responsibility (10 per cent), together with the older person's expressed wishes (6 per cent). Nevertheless, nearly half the helpers found that in time they were able to perform tasks which they did not initially think they were able or willing to do, the main ones being toileting/commode emptying (20 per cent), bathing/washing down (13 per cent), dressing and undressing (8 per cent) and getting up and putting to bed (6 per cent). A willingness to extend the range of caring activities undertaken would tend to follow the development of a relationship and personal commitment to a person. For a handful of helpers there were a few tasks which they were no longer willing or able to do. These tended to be household or social activities such as preparation

**Table 4.10**

*Difficulties met by helper in supporting the older person*

| Area of difficulty | % |
| --- | --- |
| Difficult personality/personality clash | 39 |
| Nature of illness, extent of frailty | 26 |
| Older person's reluctance to accept help | 21 |
| Older person's confusion | 21 |
| Problems with formal carers/agency | 17 |
| Arguments (with older person/carers) over money management | 16 |
| Incontinence | 14 |
| Problems with informal carers | 14 |
| Deafness, communication difficulties | 13 |
| Dirty home conditions | 13 |
| Situation too worrying/too much responsibility | 12 |
| Inappropriate housing, mobility/access problems | 11 |
| Impoverished, ill equipped home | 8 |
| Uncertainty about tasks/help required | 8 |
| Travelling problems/distance | 7 |
| Number of helpers = 119 | |

of meals and drinks and telephone calls to the older person. The latter could be a natural reaction to excess demands being made. Eleven per cent of helpers actually gave up working with one or more older people, a further 7 per cent having seriously considered giving up.

In the light of the care managers need to control helper workload, 71 per cent of all helpers had never felt that unreasonable demands had been placed on them. However, such demands were quite frequent in 10 per cent of cases, the most common source of pressure being from the older person (16 per cent of these). Nine per cent of helpers experienced pressure from their own feelings of worry or responsibility for the older person. A similar number felt the pressure was applied by the care managers, and pointed to a general excess of commitments.

Importantly, for those few helpers experiencing undue pressure, half had found these problems had been usually resolved, and most others had found them partially resolved. Nearly all had discussed their problems with the care manager.

### The clustering of rewards

As with the analysis of motivations, after examining individual rewards, patterns of rewards were considered. By performing a cluster analysis (Romesburg, 1984) based upon the twelve types of rewards, the 119 helpers distributed themselves most naturally between nine groups. Of these, one contained only three helpers, two contained two helpers, and one contained one

UNIVERSITY OF WINCHESTER
LIBRARY

helper. Because of their small size, these four groups were ignored. The characteristics of the remaining five groups are now considered in turn.

*Group 1 — usefulness/time to spare/independence* This group of nineteen helpers felt rewarded over a wide range of factors. Nearly all (95 per cent) were located in the outer districts, with a high proportion of helpers who found the work gave them something to do and filled in their time (84 per cent) as well as providing a sense of purpose (100 per cent), this group corresponds to the usefulness/time to spare cluster of Qureshi et al. (1989). In addition, the very high proportion of helpers deriving greater personal independence (95 per cent) compared with the mean of only 37 per cent, meant that this group also showed similarities to the independence/stimulation cluster (Qureshi et al., 1989). These helpers also experienced rewards from an improvement in the older person's welfare (100 per cent), a respect/attachment to them (95 per cent), being needed (100 per cent), an enjoyment of responsibility (84 per cent), improved social life (79 per cent) and a development of their own education or skills (84 per cent). Very few ever considered leaving the scheme and over two-thirds (68 per cent) felt that working for the scheme had changed their outlook on life.

This group had usually wanted to meet people (82 per cent) and to repay help received (38 per cent).

*Group 2 — usefulness* This constituted the largest group of helpers (67). Nearly half (47 per cent) wanted to use their skills/knowledge and 94 per cent wanted a chance to be useful. Nearly all (96 per cent) were rewarded by the older person's gratitude and by their attachment to them. All helpers derived a sense of achievement. However, none were rewarded by an improved social life and only one helper in five (21 per cent) felt they had developed their own knowledge or skills.

*Group 3 — payment* Almost three-quarters of these fifteen helpers had joined the scheme in order to earn some money. Only about half were attracted by the scheme as an interest outside the home and only one helper in three by the desire to meet people. Few felt the work would repay help received, none felt it would take their mind off their own worries, and few saw it as experience for a job or career. Only in two instances did they feel it would use their skills or knowledge and only one helper in five saw it as a social obligation.

Regarding the rewards they obtained from the work, only about half felt this was due to an improvement in the older person's welfare, and none obtained a sense of achievement. Only two had cent obtained career experience and achieved greater personal independence, and only one felt their own education or skills had been developed. Two had left or considered leaving the scheme due to too much pressure, but none had left because of alternative employment.

*Group 4 — human capital building* Of this small group of six helpers, only one was motivated by a desire to fill spare time or obtain stimulation, and only one saw it as a means of using their skills or knowledge, however four saw it as a social obligation.

Of the rewards obtained, all these helpers were pleased by an improvement in the welfare of the older person, and saw it as career experience. All but one saw it as a development of their own education or skills. In contrast, only one helper was rewarded by the older person's gratitude or appreciation, and none derived an enjoyment of responsibility or found it acted as a time filler. All helpers felt that the scheme had been an important part of their life.

*Group 5 — leavers group* This group of only four helpers had on average been employed by the scheme for only four weeks at the time of interview. Their mean age (47) was a little higher than the average (41). All had resigned, 3 having insufficient work and two having relationship problems with the older person. Most of the group had seen the scheme as an interest outside the home and as an opportunity both to help someone in need, and to look after someone. The wish to earn money was not common. A half were motivated by a wish to take their mind of their own worries. These showed similarities to the so called 'diversion therapy group' of Qureshi et al. (1989) who also had a high drop-out rate. Three out of the four helpers were rewarded by finding the work 'something to do'.

## Motivation and rewards — the experience of helpers

If providing a setting that presents the probability of attracting suitable helpers is necessary for recruitment, then ensuring that the setting generates appropriate rewards is important for retaining helpers. Here, the relationship between the two is considered. In this section an examination is made of the relationships between people's motivations, rewards and whether or not they continued as helpers.

### The relationship between motivations and their corresponding rewards

The relationship between motivations and corresponding rewards is shown in Table 4.11 by means of correlation. It can be seen that the correlation coefficients are rather low except in the cases of 'time to spare' (0.34) and 'career experience' (0.42). The large negative correlation (-0.30) regarding pay is presumably due to the fact that the helpers who were the most motivated to receive pay were also the most likely to be critical over the level of pay. In contrast, the motivations and rewards selected by Qureshi et al. (1989) in the Kent study all have correlations of between 0.41 and 0.72. The lower Gateshead values were in part attributable to rather more helpers receiving a particular

**Table 4.11**

*Relationship between motivations and rewards*

| Motivation | Reward | Receiving reward % | Pearson Correlation Coefficient |
|---|---|---|---|
| *Social contact* | | | |
| To meet people | Respect for/emotional attachment to older person | 86 | 0.27 |
| To fill up spare time/provide stimulation | Something to do/filling in time | 49 | 0.34 |
| To meet people | Improved social life/meeting others | 18 | 0.24 |
| *Esteem needs* | | | |
| A chance to do something useful, to give something | Sense of purpose/worthwhile activity | 97 | -0.047 |
| It's an interest outside the home, separate identity | Greater personal independence | 37 | 0.049 |
| To earn some money | Greater personal independence | 37 | 0.014 |
| It's an interest outside the home, separate identity | Improved social life/meeting others | 37 | 0.25 |
| To repay help received as I've had good fortune | Greater personal independence | 37 | 0.17 |
| *Material needs* | | | |
| To earn some money | Pay received is sufficient | 74 | -0.30 |
| Experience for a job/career | Career experience/professional contact | 40 | 0.42 |
| Experience for a job/career | Development of own education/ skills | 35 | 0.11 |
| *Altruism-personality* | | | |
| To look after, or care for someone | Improvement in older person's welfare/quality of life | 86 | 0.026 |
| To help someone in need | Feelings of indispensability/being needed by older person | 84 | 0.057 |
| Number of helpers = 116 | | | |

reward than were expressing the corresponding motivations. Thus, although only 25 per cent expressed the wish to obtain experience for a job or career (human capital building), 41 per cent were rewarded by such experience. The same argument applies in the case of time to spare and usefulness. Thus expectations were lower than experience.

In the case of affiliation, it is clear from Table 4.12 that most people anticipating improved social contacts did not experience this in practice. Moreover, most of those looking for an interest outside the home or separate identity did not achieve greater personal independence. In the case of time to spare, affiliation and human capital building, a helper was much more likely to receive one of these three rewards when the corresponding motivation had already been expressed. Thus 76 per cent of helpers motivated by human capital building were so rewarded, while only 29 per cent of these not so motivated were

**Table 4.12**
*Proportions for whom motivations are also rewards*

| Motivation | Total number | Reward received | |
|---|---|---|---|
| | | Number | % |
| *Time to spare:* | | | |
| motivation expressed | 37 | 27 | 73 |
| motivation not expressed | 79 | 29 | 37 |
| *Affiliation:* | | | |
| motivation expressed | 68 | 17 | 25 |
| motivation not expressed | 48 | 3 | 6 |
| *Human capital building:* | | | |
| motivation expressed | 29 | 22 | 76 |
| motivation not expressed | 87 | 25 | 29 |
| *Usefulness:* | | | |
| motivation expressed | 107 | 104 | 97 |
| motivation not expressed | 9 | 9 | 100 |
| *Independence:* | | | |
| motivation expressed | 81 | 32 | 40 |
| motivation not expressed | 35 | 12 | 34 |
| *Payment:* | | | |
| motivation expressed | 57 | 34 | 60 |
| motivation not expressed | 59 | 51 | 86 |
| Number of helpers = 116 | | | |

rewarded. However, this result did not emerge for the remaining three motivations tabulated. Indeed the rather smaller proportion of cases rewarded by adequate pay from the group who were motivated by pay is a result of the negative association between this motivation and reward which has already been commented upon.

In Table 4.13 the association between two types of altruistic motivation and two types of satisfaction as rewards have been investigated. Helpers expressing feelings of altruism can be divided into those who want to look after others through personally looking after them (altruistic personality), and those who are simply wishing to improve life for older people (empathetic altruism). On the rewards side there are those who gain satisfaction because they had a personal hand in successful caring (contribution satisfaction), and those gaining satisfaction simply because of an improvement in the older person's quality of life (client state satisfaction). It can be seen that in each combination of motivation and reward, most helpers expressing the motivation were rewarded. The proportion not expressing the motivation who were rewarded was in each case only slightly less. The proportions of helpers in each group are fairly

**Table 4.13**

*Satisfaction and altruism: associations between 'contribution satisfaction',[a] 'client state satisfaction',[b] 'altruistic personality',[c] and 'empathetic altruism'[d]*

|  | Total number | Reward received | |
|---|---|---|---|
|  |  | Number | % |
| *Motivation – altruistic personality*[c] | | | |
| *Reward – contribution satisfaction:*[a] | | | |
| motivation expressed | 97 | 80 | 82 |
| motivation not expressed | 19 | 15 | 79 |
| *Motivation – altruistic personality*[c] | | | |
| *Reward – client state satisfaction:*[b] | | | |
| motivation expressed | 97 | 84 | 87 |
| motivation not expressed | 19 | 16 | 84 |
| *Motivation – empathetic altruism*[d] | | | |
| *Reward – contribution satisfaction:*[a] | | | |
| motivation expressed | 91 | 75 | 82 |
| motivation not expressed | 25 | 20 | 80 |
| *Motivation – empathetic altruism*[d] | | | |
| *Reward – client state satisfaction:*[b] | | | |
| motivation expressed | 91 | 79 | 87 |
| motivation not expressed | 25 | 21 | 84 |

Number of helpers = 116

a Sense of own achievement in successful caring.
b Improvement in older person's welfare/quality of life.
c To look after or care for someone.
d To work with the elderly.

similar whichever combination of motivation and reward is chosen. Much less divergence between expectation and reward was identified than was the case for Qureshi et al. (1989) in Kent.

### Sustained involvement and drop-out of helpers

Rewards were likely to be a critical element in determining turnover of those working for the scheme, and it is noteworthwy that 62 per cent never considered leaving. Ten per cent had occasionally thought of leaving, and of those interviewed 23 per cent had already left. The reasons for resigning or for considering leaving were multiple. The most common cause was a change in some personal/family circumstances (13 per cent), though this nearly always seemed to be in combination with feelings of some type of dissatisfaction with the work. Eleven per cent of helpers left in order to take up alternative employment, though this also was generally combined with problems with the work. Finding another job was sometimes in response to dissatisfaction with work as a helper. The remaining reasons for wishing to leave were all direct problems. Eight per cent of helpers complained of insufficient pay and 7 per cent of insufficient work, while a similar proportion were under too much pressure.

For the 33 helpers who had already left, 30 of them stated that they would have liked to continue with the scheme had circumstances permitted. Although leaving would sometimes have been due to a change in circumstances unconnected with the scheme, like the family having to move away because of the husband's job, others would have due to inadequate pay and still others because of difficulties in the relationship with particular individuals.

Turning to the helpers who had not left, all but two envisaged continuing for as long as necessary with their current older people, suggesting a substantial commitment to known individuals. Moreover, nearly all would have liked work with new people had their existing work come to an end, indicating an overall commitment to the scheme. Forty per cent of all helpers felt that working for the scheme had influenced their views and 76 per cent found working for the scheme constituted an important part of their life. Thirty-nine per cent had learnt more about older people while a further 13 per cent had developed a more positive view of older people. Only two individuals had developed more negative views.

*Motivations, rewards, drop-out and dislike of the work* There was not a lot of evidence for a close association between each motivation and its corresponding reward. Nevertheless, helpers wanting to fill their spare time were likely to be successful in doing this, and helpers wanting to be useful found a sense of purpose in the work. Also helpers wanting an interest outside the home or a separate identity tended to find their pay reasonable, they had successfully achieved a measure of independence.

Two main groups emerged. The first of these was characterised by a fulfilled need to be altruistic, while the second, characterised by human capital building, was associated with a greater likelihood of leaving the scheme. This ties in with 11 per cent of all helpers (or nearly half of those who dropped out) having left the scheme to take up alternative employment.

*Factors associated with the drop-out of helpers from the scheme* It would clearly be useful to know at the point of the initial recruitment of helpers the circumstances that are likely to favour sustained involvement, together with causes of helper drop-out. An attempt was therefore made to identify the different characteristics that are associated with staying or drop out. The method was discriminant analysis, using the following sets of information in turn:

- Information on helper characteristics available at the time of the initial interview.
- Fourteen different possible types of motivation from the initial interview.
- Twelve types of reward from follow-up interviews.

- A combination of the rewards and other advantages/difficulties of the work.

Although one reason often given for withdrawal was personal/family circumstances extraneous to the scheme, this was nearly always combined with other reasons. In view of the multiple nature of reasons it was decided that all cases should be included in the analysis.

*Using characteristics available at the time of the initial interview to predict drop-out*
Before considering the results of discriminant analysis it is worth commenting that Qureshi et al. (1983) discovered a high association between sustained involvement and previous experience with older people. This relationship was investigated for these helpers, but was found to be quite different. Of those helpers without prior experience of working with older people only 25 per cent dropped out, whilst 50 per cent of helpers with experience left. One reason for this appeared to be that helpers experienced in working with older people were more likely to be wanting experience for a career, and of these 34 per cent dropped out compared with only 23 per cent for those who were not so motivated.

The nine variables that entered the discriminant function are shown in Table 4.14. The results suggest that men were less likely to drop out, although there were few males. Owner-occupiers were more likely to sustain their involvement, and those employed part-time were less likely to drop out, whilst the unemployed were more likely to leave. The more reasons the helper specified for looking for work (i.e. job/social/voluntary), the more likely they were to drop out. Those of skilled manual status were also more likely to drop out. Understandably, the longer a helper had been working for the scheme, the more likely they were to drop-out since the probability of other events intervening was greater.

*Using helper motivations to predict drop-out* The motivations predicting drop-our are shown in Table 4.15. It can be seen that those wanting to look after, or care for someone (altruistic personality) were more likely to drop out, while those wanting to do something useful or to give something more often sustained their involvement. Also, helpers who were already involved with the work were more likely to drop out.

*Using helper rewards to predict drop-out* The rewards predicting drop-out are shown in Table 4.16. Those who experienced the appreciativeness or gratitude of the older person were less likely to drop out. Those who had obtained career experience or professional contact more frequently dropped out, as a result of obtaining employment. However, when the reward was the development of helper's own education or skills, and thus not a means to obtaining a job, helpers were much more likely to sustain their involvement. Once again, helpers who had been working longer for the scheme were more likely to have dropped out.

**Table 4.14**
*Predicting drop-out in terms of helper characteristics*

| Characteristic | Coefficient |
| --- | --- |
| Gender (whether female) | 2.20 |
| Owner-occupier | -1.04 |
| Employed part-time at time of recruitment | -1.23 |
| Unemployed at time of recruitment | 1.34 |
| Was looking mainly for a job/career related experience | 0.86 |
| Was looking mainly for social activity | 0.93 |
| Was looking mainly for voluntary work | 0.90 |
| Skilled manual status | 0.93 |
| Number of weeks working for scheme | 0.0052 |
| Constant | -8.16 |

| | Actual group | Predicted group | |
| --- | --- | --- | --- |
| | | Stay % | Leave % |
| Wilks' lambda = 0.64442 | | | |
| F = 6.7 | | | |
| df = 9,109 | | | |
| p value <0.001 | Stay % | 73.3 | 26.7 |
| Correct predictions = 79% | Leave % | 6.1 | 93.9 |
| Number of helpers = 119 | | | |

**Table 4.15**
*Predicting drop-out in terms of helper motivations*

| Motivation | Coefficient |
| --- | --- |
| A chance to do something useful, to give something | -1.16 |
| To look after, or care for someone | 1.71 |
| Already doing the work, but offer of pay was helpful | -1.73 |
| Number of weeks working for scheme | 0.0060 |
| Constant | -3.61 |

| | Actual group | Predicted group | |
| --- | --- | --- | --- |
| | | Stay % | Leave % |
| Wilks' lambda = 0.76334 | | | |
| F = 8.5 | | | |
| df = 4,100 | | | |
| p value <0.001 | Stay % | 62.8 | 37.2 |
| Correct predictions = 71% | Leave % | 3.4 | 96.6 |
| Number of helpers = 119 | | | |

**Table 4.16**
*Predicting drop-out in terms of helper rewards*

| Reward | | Coefficient | |
|---|---|---|---|
| Appreciativeness/gratitude of older person | | -0.90 | |
| Career experience/professional contact | | 0.78 | |
| Development of own education/skills | | -1.35 | |
| Number of weeks working for scheme | | 0.0057 | |
| Constant | | -2.25 | |
| Wilks' lambda = 0.78153 | *Actual group* | *Predicted group* | |
| F = 8.0 | | *Stay %* | *Leave %* |
| df = 4,114 | | | |
| p value <0.001 | Stay % | 62.8 | 37.2 |
| Correct predictions = 70% | Leave % | 12.1 | 87.9 |
| Number of helpers = 119 | | | |

*Using helper rewards and other advantages and problems of the work to predict drop-out* The factors describing other rewards and advantages which predicted drop-out are shown in Table 4.17.

Helpers receiving 'altruism-personality' and 'human capital building' rewards were more likely to drop out. The first of these results was unexpected, though it is unsurprising that helpers who obtained career experience would subsequently tend to drop out so that their careers could be furthered. It was found that the larger the number of helper contacts with the care manager, the more likely the helper was to drop out. Presumably helpers who sustain their involvement were more able to get on with the work on their own without needing the support of the care manager. Moreover helpers who felt they had had sufficient contact with the care manager were less likely to drop out.

Helpers who felt that the demands placed on them by the scheme were unreasonable were more likely to drop out. Also helpers who found they were performing tasks which they would prefer not to, through assuming excess responsibility, tended to drop out more frequently. These were the helpers who became over-involved.

The helpers who performed a wide variety of household tasks, personal care tasks or tasks responding to social or emotional needs were less likely to drop out.

Those helpers experiencing problems with formal carers or agencies were more likely to sustain their involvement. This surprising result may arise because those who left did not become as involved with agencies. Difficulties over money management with older people or their carers also led to helpers dropping out.

**Table 4.17**
*Predicting drop-out in terms of helper rewards and other advantages and problems*

| Reward, advantage, problem | Coefficient |
|---|---|
| Feelings of indispensability/being needed by elderly person | 1.13 |
| Career experience/professional contact | 1.03 |
| Annual number of contacts with the care manager | 0.0021 |
| Helper has had sufficient contact with the care manager | -1.15 |
| Demands placed on helper by scheme unreasonable | 1.39 |
| Self-pressure applied due to own assessment of need/feelings of worry/responsibility | 0.97 |
| Number of types of household tasks tackled | -0.43 |
| Number of types of personal care tasks tackled | -0.19 |
| Number of types of social/emotional needs tackled | -0.19 |
| Problems with formal carers/agency | -0.76 |
| Arguments over money management (with elderly person/carers) | 0.66 |
| Number of weeks working for scheme | 0.0059 |
| Constant | -0.97 |

| | Actual group | Predicted group | |
|---|---|---|---|
| | | Stay % | Leave % |
| Wilks' lambda = 0.44174 | | | |
| F = 11.1 | | | |
| df = 12,105 | | | |
| p value <0.001 | Stay % | 88.4 | 11.6 |
| Correct predictions = 90% | Leave % | 6.3 | 93.8 |
| Number of helpers = 119 | | | |

## Motivations and rewards

At times helpers appeared to have received rewards beyond their original motivations. Indeed, most of those who were motivated by the desire to help were rewarded by the satisfaction gained through this. A particularly common cause of drop out from the scheme was change in the personal circumstances of helpers themselves. Those with motivations associated with socially useful activity were more likely to remain involved, whereas those wishing to express a personal caring need were more likely to drop out. Those with previous caring experience were more likely to leave, since such individuals could more readily move into the range of labour market activities associated with care, such as nursing homes and home help provision. Hence it would seem that, from the perspective of those providing a service, the advantages conferred through recruiting individuals with previous caring experience have to be traded against the greater probability of such individuals finding alternative employment. Stability and continuity of care was provided more by those seeking useful activity, than by those motivated by a more personality-related desire to help.

### Helpers from different areas

Another factor influencing the availability of local help is the characteristics of the local area. The scheme was undertaken in both the outer and inner city areas with some different patterns of helper recruitment and utilisation in each. The outer area was a relatively stable and traditional working class district, though with a significant number of people from the middle classes, not dissimilar from the 'Sunnyside' described by Abrams (Bulmer, 1986). The inner city was a more working class district. The care managers commented on the differences that faced them in raising support and help for older people with similar problems in these two districts, reflected in the different availability of potential helpers.

Of the helpers interviewed, 74 worked in the outer city district where the scheme was first introduced. The other 45 came from a geographically separate district in the inner city, the scheme's second operational area. The inner city area was deprived and still dominated by old, privately rented terraced housing, but with some council redevelopment and pre-war owner-occupied housing. The outer city was an amalgamation of established urban districts and villages absorbed into the metropolitan borough boundaries in 1974. It contained large areas of post war council housing, and of owner occupied, suburban housing, and was altogether a more mixed area. Being on the edge of the borough, the outer city area attracted migration out from the inner city, as well as having a substantial indigenous population.

The helpers were thus recruited from two different socio-economic contexts, but worked in a similar practice and organisational setting. They were all recruited by the same care managers with the same objectives and underlying values. The majority of helpers in each area were working class, although in the inner city it was a higher proportion.

In their review of Good Neighbour Schemes in England, Abrams et al. (1981) showed that 'schemes develop most readily in areas where there is a large supply of people (mainly women) who not only do not do full-time work but can also afford to meet the costs involved in being a good neighbour' (p.37). The greater incidence which they found of schemes in prosperous regions of the country indicated that good neighbour schemes tend to flourish 'where need and a certain level of prosperity exist side by side' (p.38). Thus there would seem to be some evidence of an inverse relationship between inner urban areas and the potential for informal care. Indeed, it had often been argued that neighbouring is a declining feature of urban society particularly in the inner areas (Keller, 1968; Key, 1965). Notwithstanding this, traditional British community studies have tended to argue that patterns of neighbouring and social support thrive in inner areas (Young and Willmott, 1957). Such an argument has also been advanced by Collins and Pancoast (1976) who did, however, indicate that dwellers in urban environments tend to participate in more loose-knit networks.

It is perhaps this difference in the nature or quality of social networks rather than their extensiveness which may differentiate the inner urban environment from other areas. Abrams (1984) compared two good neighbour schemes in two distinctly different areas. The one, 'Sunnyside', was a relatively stable working class district with a traditional system of kinship support providing substantial care for older people. The other, 'Alphaville', was a mixed area close to the centre of the city, although containing a substantial middle class, and could be described as a zone of transition. Abrams noted important differences between the two schemes reflecting differences in the informal networks in the two areas.

Similarly, a large number of differences were observed between the outer city and the inner city regarding the helpers' experience of the scheme. The helpers in the inner city were somewhat older, with fewer children at home and more often had paid employment. They were more likely to be recruited through a newspaper advertisement, a common channel for those seeking paid employment generally.

There was more work available to helpers in the inner city. The greater ease in geographically matching helpers with older people in this more concentrated urban area undoubtedly played a part in this. They were less likely to have to wait before work became available, and spent more days and hours per week in working for the scheme. They were more likely to have worked continuously and less likely to have found a lack of regular employment difficult. However, one problem associated with this extra availability of work was that inner city helpers were more likely to experience pressure due to an excess of commitment, and indeed more often left or considered leaving because of this. They were more likely to have given up with an older person, and those helpers who dropped out had no further contact with them. However, one reason for the inner city helpers having more work was that the majority were dependent on the extra income this brought in. Care managers were therefore obliged to keep their inner city helpers busy, otherwise they were likely to leave. The research reported by Abrams is relevant here. In discussing one of the few neighbourhood care schemes which employed paid carers, he pointed out that money may be a necessary facilitator for working class people to provide care for their neighbours:

> Stonegate's paid carers were all middle-aged and over, mostly from old inner city areas so that they had experienced traditional neighbourliness while in general they felt that being a warden or a home help was something they knew about, could do, and would like, but payment was

necessary to generate and harness their neighbourly talents because of their need to take a job. (Bulmer, 1986, p.180).

The parallels with this are particularly strong in the Gateshead inner city area, where helpers displayed a strong sense of commitment to looking after frail older people and anticipated personal satisfaction from doing it, but often had to give personal priority to earning money. A lower proportion of helpers in the outer city expressed this priority.

The nature of housing was rather different in the inner city. There was a smaller proportion of owner-occupiers amongst the helpers themselves. Aspects of the older people's housing were also different. Activities associated with lighting and maintaining a fire, although frequent in the outer city, rarely occurred in the inner city. Although this was presumably a result of a greater proportion of older people in local authority accommodation, this did not mean improved conditions. On the contrary, helpers were more likely to have experienced dirty home conditions, and impoverished ill-equipped homes. Nevertheless, this type of housing was less likely to be inappropriate and mobility or access problems were less frequent.

The informal network in the inner city appeared to be weaker. Here the helpers were never recruited through the older person's informal network and it was less likely that the person they first helped was known to them. Friends and neighbours appeared to be less frequently involved in helping them (Snow, 1981). Equally, contact between helpers for general mutual support or guidance was much less frequent, and it followed that such contact less often improved the social life of the helper. The weaker nature of the informal network in the inner city area is similar to the findings of Abrams et al. (1981) in their review of Good Neighbour Schemes discussed above.

Contact with the care manager did not appear to compensate for this weak informal network. In fact fewer helpers had regular contact with the care manager, and helpers relied less on their direction or support generally. Nonetheless, for some inner city helpers, the reliance on the care manager had increased since the helper first started work and received higher levels of emotional and moral support; this was not the case for any of the helpers located in the outer city.

Only slightly more of the inner city helpers, (60 per cent as opposed to 54 per cent) said they wanted a job but there were major differences between the numbers wanting a social outlet (65 per cent in the outer city, 18 per cent in the inner city), or voluntary work (40 per cent in outer city, 20 per cent in inner city). The numbers looking for a career-based activity were similar (15 per cent and 14 per cent). This suggests that the outer city helpers were motivated by a greater variety of objectives than the inner city helpers, or were more open-minded about what sort of activity they took up.

Although helpers from both areas had been searching for a personal outlet or a new interest, which would bring them a sense of personal fulfilment, this tendency was particularly strong in the outer city. Here, many helpers, although committed to the care of their families, found their domestic role was insufficiently fulfilling on its own. They wanted to supplement it with something outside the home, which would give their lives new interest and variety. The theme of community involvement motivated significantly more helpers in the outer city. They also more frequently expressed the need to care for someone.

It may be that the reasons why this search for self-expression outside the family appeared to figure more prominently in the outer city than in the inner city are linked with earlier observations about helper's need for money. Fewer helpers in the outer city seemed beset by immediate financial need and more of them could afford to think in terms of self-fulfilment and take time to look around until they found an outlet which offered them the personal returns they wanted, with or without substantial material gain. In the inner city, more helpers had to give priority to getting paid work, often as much of it as they could fit in. They attached importance to the work being worthwhile and satisfying, but could not afford to give priority to self-fulfilment. Inner city helpers often referred to themselves and their colleagues as being essentially very busy people.

There were distinct differences of emphasis between inner city and outer city helpers regarding the factors which motivated them, although, in individual cases, there was a great deal of overlap. Overall, the outer city helpers voiced a much broader range of motivations. In both areas, many helpers were quite keen to earn money, and saw their work primarily as a paid job. In both areas, helpers made clear their attraction to useful caring. The outer city helpers, however, also placed considerable emphasis on their desire for personal fulfilment, social encounters and community involvement. A greater number expressed a need to meet people, to provide help and to satisfy a desire for social giving.

This suggests a picture of outer city helpers having more time on their hands, and more inclination or opportunity to think in terms of their intellectual and social development, and of the contribution they should make to the wider community. Inner city helpers seemed to be more pressurised in terms of time, energy, and finance. They had a deep emotional drive towards caring and were clear about the personal satisfaction which looking after someone would offer them but they did not so readily broaden their aspirations to talk about personal or community development. They believed in the work, and they got on with it. Outer city helpers tended to be more steadily paced and thoughtful, with a greater tendency to intellectualise about the caring role in society, and the role they would like to play. There was a difference of style and emphasis, and a difference in how helpers perceived themselves in relation to the people they sought to help. To what extent can these two groups be differentiated?

*Differences in the characteristics of inner city and outer city helpers*

Table 4.18 shows the items most likely to identify whether a helper was situated in the inner city or outer city. Logistic regression was used to attempt to differentiate these helpers. The predictor variables were drawn from a pool that included background details of the helper, financial circumstances, the type of work they were looking for at the time of application, their motivations, experience of the scheme and rewards.

It can be seen that helpers in the outer city were more likely to have children under seventeen living at home and be owner-occupiers. Although residents in the outer city area were generally better off, more helpers in this area received state benefits. Nevertheless, it was the inner city helpers who were slightly more likely to be looking mainly for a job or career related experience when they applied to join the scheme. The rather broader range of aims

**Table 4.18**
*Differences in the characteristics of inner city and outer city helpers*

|  | Coefficient | p value |
|---|---|---|
| **Basic details** | | |
| Children under 17 at home | 9.80 | 0.03 |
| Owner occupier | 11.23 | 0.02 |
| Receipt of state benefits | 6.74 | 0.04 |
| **Type of work sought** | | |
| Job/career-related experience | -3.36 | 0.17 |
| Social activity | 5.67 | 0.01 |
| Voluntary work | 5.44 | 0.04 |
| Any with comparable pay and conditions | 5.24 | 0.01 |
| **Motivation for joining scheme** | | |
| To help someone in need | 7.95 | 0.02 |
| Take mind off own worries | 5.28 | 0.04 |
| **Experience of scheme** | | |
| Work coincided largely with expectations | -5.99 | 0.03 |
| More or less continuous work | -7.86 | 0.01 |
| Enough contact with care manager | -7.95 | 0.08 |
| **Rewards of scheme** | | |
| Enjoyment of taking responsibility | 7.96 | 0.01 |
| Something to do to fill in time | 6.90 | 0.03 |
| Greater personal independence | 14.02 | 0.01 |
| Constant | -17.34 | 0.01 |
| Lave's adjusted R squared = 0.89 | | |
| Correct predictions = 96% | | |
| Number of helpers = 119 | | |

characterising helpers from the outer city is confirmed by their also looking for some kind of social activity or voluntary work. Despite the impression that helpers in the outer city were better off and could afford to be more selective in their choice of job, it turned out that significantly more of these helpers would have taken any job with comparable pay and conditions. Helpers in the outer city were more often motivated by a wish to help someone in need reflecting a caring identity more likely to be prevalent in a relatively more affluent area. Outer city helpers were also more likely to see the work as a means of taking their minds off their own worries and were more likely to have been without work before applying to join the scheme.

Because inner city helpers applied to the scheme primarily as a job, it is perhaps unsurprising that their experience of the scheme was closer to their expectations than in the outer city, where helpers had a wider range of aims to be satisfied. Because inner city helpers had more work from the scheme, there were less likely to be breaks since being appointed. Helpers in the outer city were more likely to be dissatisfied with the amount of contact with the care manager. They may have seen this type of contact as an attraction of the scheme, particularly those who wanted to take their minds off their own worries. Despite this, outer city helpers were more likely to have been rewarded by having something to do to fill their time and greater personal independence, as well as the enjoyment of responsibility. Thus overall this analysis helps to confirm the differences between the helpers in the two areas which had previously emerged.

### Differences in patterns of helping between inner and outer city helpers

Analysis of the tasks undertaken also indicates some differences between helpers. Those in the inner city were more likely to be focused on basic care tasks, such as toileting, housework, bedmaking and washing. Those in the outer district, conversely, undertook a wider range of activities, including regular check ups, managing medication, day sitting and dealing with business letters as well as basic care tasks. Again, helping the older person with handicraft or leisure activities was much more frequent in the outer city, where they were more frequently helped to improve their mobility. Nearly twice the proportion of helpers in the inner city cared for at least one confused older person. It was therefore unsurprising that the inner city helpers were more frequently involved in most aspects of reality orientation, and had more frequent contact with the care manager.

Although joint visits with the district nurse were made only in the inner city, helpers here had much less contact with home helps. Contacts with the older person's family, neighbours or friends were more frequent in the inner city, this contact being mainly in person, but also to a lesser degree by telephone or written note. Contact usually took the form of routinely keeping in touch.

Interestingly, this fails to confirm the earlier observation that informal networks were generally weaker in the inner city.

## Conclusions

As has been seen, helpers proved to be a key element in care managers' strategy to provide more user-centred community care. They were the main resource that could be directly influenced by care managers, so as to act more responsively and flexibly, providing care at times and in ways that were more appropriate. These arrangements may represent one way in which purchasing social services departments may seek to extend the flexibility of domiciliary care (Leat and Ungerson, 1994). Hence, aspects of helpers' roles and their work in the scheme have been an important part of this study.

Most helpers were aged between 30 and 50 years of age and were female. Their motivations for participating in the scheme were multiple, involving a combination of financial and personal factors leading them to balance these elements in a personal calculus of benefit and loss. These different balances of motivations and rewards were reflected in the different circumstances of different helpers, the tasks they undertook, the satisfactions and difficulties of helping, and the likelihood of their continuing in this caring role. There were also clear differences in these factors between helpers in the different social contexts of the inner city and more outlying areas.

The linkage between helper characteristics, motivations, rewards and subsequent 'careers' is of practical relevance to the development of a mixed economy of community support. Ungerson (1993) has noted that such forms of 'work' and 'pay' are attractive to many women who give their services to care in often difficult and demanding circumstances. As a consequence, blurring the worlds of work and care has some value to those engaged in it. Evers (1994) has suggested that this requires reframing the position of such care-giving activity away from discussion of threats to traditional care-giving through marketisation towards the perception of such blurring processes as an opportunity. He suggests, of paid caring, that:

> The payments can be conceived as part of a broader package of resources and infrastructures needed for a truly developmental policy, instead of a policy which colonises the existing institutions of volunteering and family care (p.39).

# 5  Responding to Particular Needs

The previous chapter described the process of care management in the scheme and the helpers recruited to it, but describing the pattern of activities provides only part of the picture. The care scheme was designed to tackle more effectively problems that are often associated with the breakdown of care in the community. This was to be achieved through more flexible and individually tailored responses to need. This chapter examines the ways in which the scheme provided care to older people with different needs. Six need or problem areas were identified and these are described below.

## Need areas

Any form of categorisation of cases by particular problems is inevitably difficult since the problems of frail older people are multiple (Bergmann, 1973). Perhaps the simplest and best-known categorisation are the 'Giants of Geriatrics' identified by Isaacs (1981), namely the four 'Is': 'Immobility', 'Incontinence', 'Instability' and 'Intellectual Impairment'. These categories were used as a basis for the analyses. To these may be added a fifth 'I', 'Informal Carers', and also the presence of depression. These six categories are shown in Box 5.1 and each is considered in turn. They cannot, of course, be seen as mutually exclusive categories, and the majority of the older people experienced need in two or three of the areas.

The care manager activities undertaken overall and with each sub group are shown in Table 5.1. This is based upon information gathered at case reviews. The percentages are shown for all cases, as well as broken down by the different need categories. These are discussed in the relevant sections below.

It is important to note that in this chapter we are focusing on an analysis of process, to understand service responses to different problems. In this analysis

---

**Box 5.1**
*The six categories of problem areas*

| | |
|---|---|
| Immobility | Needing help in getting in or out of bed or chair |
| Instability | Frequent risk of falling |
| Incontinence | Frequently incontinent of urine or faeces |
| Impaired | Moderately/severely confused |
| Depressed | Moderately/severely depressed |
| Informal carer stress | Carer scoring 5 or more on the malaise scale |

---

all cases receiving the scheme have been included, since the focus is upon the scheme as a whole and not just the matched pairs. Consequently, differences between experimental and comparison groups may be seen which have been eliminated in the matching process. In the following sections aspects of need, cost and outcomes are presented for each need category. Where costs are presented a 1981-2 price base is employed. The costing approach is described in Chapter 8.

*Immobility*

The effects of immobility on activities of daily living will have wide-ranging consequences, so that difficulties with dressing or making a hot drink can be considered alongside problems of walking, getting in and out of a chair or being bedfast. For example, 44 per cent needed help with transfer or were bedfast. The most physically dependent people on the scheme were bedfast. Unless such people have a great deal of family support, they are usually unable to remain at home. Through careful cooperation and shared working with the community nursing service, it proved possible to develop effective support strategies. The provision of care to cover meals, medication, washing, transfers to the commode and other activities could be rationally planned for every day. In one case, because of the frequency of visits, it was possible to arrange for a previously bedfast woman to sit up in a chair for periods of the day. This helped to lessen the probability of pressure sores as well as to provide a change of surroundings to improve morale. Given more frequent help, she was able to sit up in a chair from morning until teatime, when the helper would settle her back to bed. A helper would also join in word games and complete crossword answers that the lady had solved but due to severely arthritic fingers was unable to write down. This re-engagement in social activities significantly improved her quality of life and her will to continue. In less severe cases mobility problems could go hand-in-hand with being housebound, isolated,

**Table 5.1**
*Care manager activities and contacts by type of need as a percentage of case reviews[a]*

| | All cases | Immobility | Instability | Incontinence | Impaired | Depressed | Carer stress |
|---|---|---|---|---|---|---|---|
| **Activities** | | | | | | | |
| Exploratory/(re-)assessment | 45 | 47 | 47 | 51 | 47 | 42 | 45 |
| Information/advice | 22 | 25 | 22 | 21 | 8 | 23 | 23 |
| Mobilising resources | 66 | 67 | 64 | 73 | 61 | 63 | 60 |
| Coordinating resources | 65 | 64 | 67 | 68 | 61 | 67 | 59 |
| Check-up/review visits | 90 | 93 | 91 | 90 | 93 | 88 | 89 |
| Assist with problems/decisions | 28 | 24 | 29 | 11 | 16 | 33 | 34 |
| Sustain older person | 60 | 56 | 60 | 60 | 63 | 61 | 65 |
| Sustain family/carer | 43 | 46 | 46 | 46 | 56 | 37 | 58 |
| Sustain helper | 72 | 74 | 78 | 70 | 76 | 66 | 67 |
| Advocacy | 14 | 15 | 16 | 20 | 12 | 12 | 15 |
| **Contacts** | | | | | | | |
| General practitioner | 65 | 57 | 63 | 65 | 71 | 64 | 66 |
| District nurse | 39 | 47 | 42 | 33 | 34 | 41 | 35 |
| Total number of cases | 101 | 44 | 57 | 29 | 31 | 56 | 46 |
| Total number of reviews | 357 | 133 | 206 | 93 | 106 | 202 | 160 |

a There are up to four case reviews for each older person.

neglectful of diet, and suffering from constipation, depression and low morale. For example, a service to simply provide a meal may be by no means as straightforward as it sounds. It was necessary to encourage the older person to re-acquire appetite and to keep a check to ensure that their fluid intake was adequate. Sometimes, something as simple as re-instituting an old pattern of sitting at a laid table could be the initial move towards a more balanced diet and daily routine. Once the person's confidence was gained a further strategy could be introduction to a day group.

The assessment would often have identified a variety of needs, such as for chiropody, for a greater degree of physical activity, and for attendance at the day hospital or other activity. It was often unlikely that simply referring to the appropriate agency would alone resolve the problem. For example, further direct input from the care manager might be needed to persuade or enable the older person to make use of the resources. In the absence of an adequate domiciliary chiropody service a housebound person might be unable to reach a clinic. Providing transport in the form of an ambulance might not be enough to overcome the person's apprehension at going out and to enable them to receive the beneficial effects of attending a day hospital. A helper using their own car and providing support could overcome this resistance. Helpers performed a variety of tasks both practical and social, including assistance with washing, dressing, and getting in and out of bed, whilst always bearing in mind the strategy of utilising the older person's abilities and avoiding undermining them. On occasions helpers were trained to use physiotherapy exercises in order to practice these with the older person to enable them to regain or retain levels of functioning.

Table 5.2 compares the characteristics of those cases who were immobile with the group as a whole. The older people considered here needed help in getting in or out of bed or chairs. They closely resembled the group with 'serious physical frailty' considered by Challis and Davies (1986). The immobile group consisted of 44 care scheme cases and 52 comparison cases. From Table 5.2, it can be seen that somewhat fewer immobile cases lived alone and rather more had relatives living with them, reflecting the difficulties of caring for this degree of dependency 'at a distance'. Moreover, a slightly higher proportion of these had a carer.

These people frequently had higher levels of difficulty in the activities of dressing, toileting, feeding and bathing and their overall dependency was, consequently, much higher. Risk of falling and breathlessness were also more prevalent. As a consequence they received more frequent contact from services. They were less frequently lonely or depressed, again perhaps reflecting the extra level of contact with services and carers. The locational outcomes of the immobile group were less favourable than for the group as a whole, fewer having remained at home after one year and more having died or entered long-term hospital care, a result also found by Challis and Davies (1986) in the Kent scheme. Due to the high dependency of this group, it was to be expected

**Table 5.2**

*Comparison of those with mobility problems with all*

| | Mobility problem cases | | All cases | |
|---|---|---|---|---|
| | Care scheme | Comparison group | Care scheme | Comparison group |
| *Descriptive material* | | | | |
| Number of cases | 44 | 52 | 101 | 144 |
| Average age (years) | 80 | 80 | 81 | 80 |
| *Gender* | | | | |
| Male | 14% | 14% | 13% | 16% |
| Female | 86% | 86% | 87% | 84% |
| *Living group* | | | | |
| Alone | 68% | 59% | 75% | 69% |
| With spouse | 14% | 8% | 13% | 9% |
| Other | 18% | 33% | 12% | 22% |
| Presence of informal carer | 75% | 81% | 71% | 72% |
| *Outcomes* | | | | |
| At home | 55% | 42% | 62% | 46% |
| Local authority home | 2% | 21% | 2% | 29% |
| Private residential/nursing home | 0% | 0% | 0% | 2% |
| Long-term hospital care | 9% | 8% | 9% | 4% |
| Died | 34% | 29% | 26% | 18% |
| Moved away | 0% | 0% | 1% | 1% |
| *Problem prevalence* | | | | |
| Immobility | 100% | 100% | 44% | 36% |
| Incontinence (frequent) | 32% | 35% | 29% | 16% |
| Cognitive impairment (moderate or severe) | 30% | 29% | 31% | 30% |
| Instability (frequent falling risk) | 70% | 63% | 56% | 35% |
| Informal carer stress | 48% | 51% | 48% | 47% |
| Breathlessness | 64% | 42% | 57% | 51% |
| Giddiness | 68% | 54% | 64% | 55% |
| Eyesight | 70% | 67% | 75% | 65% |
| Hearing | 48% | 52% | 55% | 48% |
| Frequent loneliness | 46% | 52% | 57% | 61% |
| Depression (moderate or severe) | 48% | 56% | 55% | 56% |
| Anxiety (moderate or severe) | 59% | 54% | 58% | 56% |
| ADL index (0-6) | 4.7 | 4.4 | 3.4 | 2.5 |

**Table 5.2 (continued)**

|  | Mobility problem cases | | All cases | |
|---|---|---|---|---|
|  | Care scheme | Comparison group | Care scheme | Comparison group |
| *Needing help with activities of daily living* | | | | |
| Dressing | 89% | 71% | 60% | 36% |
| Getting to/using toilet | 89% | 75% | 63% | 41% |
| Feeding self (mechanical) | 23% | 25% | 13% | 12% |
| Bathing/showering | 100% | 96% | 91% | 80% |
| Making hot drink/snack | 96% | 89% | 76% | 67% |
| Preparing hot meal | 100% | 98% | 97% | 93% |
| Number of weeks alive | 43.52 | 44.36 | 44.64 | 47.52 |
| *Resources per week* | | | | |
| Net cost to SSD | £42.13 | £27.12 | £38.97 | £28.49 |
| Hours home help | 3.90 | 1.39 | 3.68 | 1.54 |
| Cost of helpers | £18.82 | - | £16.66 | - |
| Days in day care | 0.18 | 0.16 | 0.26 | 0.18 |
| Days in LA home | 0.30 | 1.79 | 0.26 | 1.84 |
| HH as % of SSD cost | 19% | 25% | 20% | 27% |
| Scheme as % of SSD cost | 43% | - | 40% | - |
| Cost to NHS @ 5% discount | £41.55 | £26.29 | £38.66 | £17.83 |
| Visits by community nurse | 2.35 | 0.57 | 1.53 | 0.41 |
| Days as hospital in-patient | 0.84 | 0.69 | 0.75 | 0.42 |

that their costs were greater than would be expected on average. For those receiving the care scheme, it can be seen from Table 5.2 that the immobile group cost slightly more on average to the social services department (£42.13) than for all types of case (£38.97). This trend was the other way round for the comparison group cases, a result of the lower resourcing by the social services department to this client group in the inner city area. These findings were largely due to differences in the time spent in local authority residential accommodation.

The additional cost of this group to the National Health Service was slightly greater, amounting to £41.55 for the subset of care scheme cases compared with £38.66 for all care scheme cases. This higher cost of the group with mobility problems was reflected in both the community nursing and hospital in-patient costs.

Above average costs to both the social services department and National Health Service were also found by Challis and Davies (1986) in the Kent scheme for cases with a serious degree of physical frailty.

Case review material on the care scheme cases, shown in Table 5.1, suggested that the care manager's social work activities and frequency of contact with other agencies was typical of their work overall. In view of the higher physical frailty of this group it is perhaps surprising that contact with the GP was less frequent than average, but this was offset by more frequent contact with district nurses.

An example of the level of involvement of the care scheme in managing mobility problems at home is illustrated by Mr J.:

Mr J. was an elderly amputee who was referred to the scheme, requiring discharge from hospital, after having his second leg amputated. He lived alone and had very little support, his brother having moved away when Mr J. was admitted to hospital, and his sister only visiting on rare occasions. The first task was to visit him in hospital to gain his confidence and to judge whether and how it might be possible to support him at home. This took several visits and meetings with hospital medical and therapy staff. Before discharge, a home visit was made jointly with hospital occupational therapist and physiotherapist and then with social services occupational therapist, since the accommodation was unsuitable with internal steps preventing access to both the kitchen and bathroom. The house was poorly furnished and he lacked a suitable bed. Mr J. also had a small dog, for whom arrangements had to be made. Hence, there was a range of environmental problems, as well as the immediate need for care provision.

An intensive package of support was organised with helpers visiting morning, afternoon and evening and the home help service at lunchtimes, with additional visits for shopping and doing the laundry. A variety of aids were organised and adaptations made to the bed to permit Mr J. to transfer from chair to bed. The district nurse trained the helpers to change dressings for pressure sores. Occupational therapists trained helpers to assist in transfer.

After a great deal of effort, new accommodation in a bungalow was arranged, which was more physically suitable and also provided an interesting outlook. Support from the helpers made it possible for him to keep his dog, who was a valued companion. The degree of support provided and the attempts to involve him in the minutiae of decision making had a marked impact on his self care and morale. He began to take pride in his personal appearance and a considerable interest in the decoration of his home. What was important in this case was the careful attention to detail, so that not only important basic care needs were met, but also important aspects of quality of life. These included ensuring that his dog could be with him, that he could prepare and cook his own meals, that he was able to be taken out by the helpers and choose clothes and curtains for himself, and helpers would regularly place his bets for him. His quality of life was further enhanced, since, for the first time he was able to sit with his dog at the window and watch the world go by.

## Instability

Risk of falling, often in the case of socially isolated people, is frequently a cause of referral for admission to residential and nursing home care. It was identified as a serious problem for 56 per cent of those receiving the care scheme and was usually accompanied by loss of confidence, anxiety and fear of the event recurring. Environmental factors were often significant contributors to the risk of falling and it was possible to tackle these by moving mats, or pieces of furniture or by correcting the height of a chair or bed. Frequently however, more complex factors were involved. For example, illness or misuse of drugs may be associated with falls but it was sometimes necessary to work to persuade a reluctant older person to accept referral to specialist medical services. Skills training could also be important. This involved obtaining the help of a physiotherapist to demonstrate methods of getting in and out of bed more safely or even suggesting how a person could fall more safely and how to get up again. Careful planning of helper visits could provide a valuable safeguard at the more critical times of the day when falls were most likely to occur. Sometimes assistance or reassurance could ensure that the risk was reduced. This, coupled with a regular and predictable pattern of visits could reduce the worry about lying on the floor undetected and could help to prevent the concomitant risk of hypothermia and secondary damage from the 'long lie' (Hall, 1982). This was often sufficient to reduce the anxiety of the older person and those around them, making care at home more viable.

Table 5.3 compares those cases who were frequently at risk of falling with the group as a whole. A rather higher proportion than average were also immobile, suffered from giddiness and required more help with activities of daily living. However cognitive impairment was less common, though more care scheme cases than average appeared depressed. Unlike the comparison group, for whom those at risk of falling were more likely to enter homes, there was no evidence of this for the care scheme group. This again suggests that the risk factors that precipitate entry to care were effectively managed by the scheme.

It can be seen that social services department costs for cases with instability were close to the average. However National Health Service costs turned out to be substantially higher for both groups. This was mainly due to a greater number of days having been spent in hospital by this subset. The high risk of fractures in this group probably contributed to this difference. Moreover, geriatric day hospital costs worked out to be larger in the care scheme group, a result also found by Challis and Davies (1986) in the Kent scheme.

**Table 5.3**
*Comparison of those at risk of falling with all*

|  | Risk of falling cases | | All cases | |
|---|---|---|---|---|
|  | Care scheme | Comparison group | Care scheme | Comparison group |
| **Descriptive material** | | | | |
| Number of cases | 57 | 51 | 101 | 144 |
| Average age (years) | 81 | 80 | 81 | 80 |
| **Gender** | | | | |
| Male | 7% | 22% | 13% | 16% |
| Female | 93% | 78% | 87% | 84% |
| **Living group** | | | | |
| Alone | 72% | 57% | 75% | 69% |
| With spouse | 14% | 12% | 13% | 9% |
| Other | 14% | 31% | 12% | 22% |
| Presence of informal carer | 77% | 73% | 71% | 72% |
| **Outcomes** | | | | |
| At home | 60% | 33% | 62% | 46% |
| Local authority home | 2% | 31% | 2% | 29% |
| Private residential/nursing home | 0% | 2% | 0% | 2% |
| Long-term hospital care | 10% | 4% | 9% | 4% |
| Died | 28% | 26% | 26% | 18% |
| Moved away | 0% | 2% | 1% | 1% |
| **Problem prevalence** | | | | |
| Immobility | 54% | 65% | 44% | 36% |
| Incontinence (frequent) | 32% | 27% | 29% | 16% |
| Cognitive impairment (moderate or severe) | 25% | 16% | 31% | 30% |
| Instability (frequent falling risk) | 100% | 100% | 56% | 35% |
| Informal carer stress | 52% | 49% | 48% | 47% |
| Breathlessness | 65% | 57% | 57% | 51% |
| Giddiness | 77% | 57% | 64% | 55% |
| Eyesight | 84% | 71% | 75% | 65% |
| Hearing | 58% | 63% | 55% | 48% |
| Frequent loneliness | 59% | 55% | 57% | 61% |
| Depression (moderate or severe) | 63% | 61% | 55% | 56% |
| Anxiety (moderate or severe) | 58% | 67% | 58% | 56% |
| ADL index (0-6) | 3.7 | 4.0 | 3.4 | 2.5 |

**Table 5.3 (continued)**

|  | Risk of falling cases | | All cases | |
|---|---|---|---|---|
|  | Care scheme | Comparison group | Care scheme | Comparison group |
| **Needing help with activities of daily living** | | | | |
| Dressing | 67% | 65% | 60% | 36% |
| Getting to/using toilet | 72% | 71% | 63% | 41% |
| Feeding self (mechanical) | 17% | 29% | 13% | 12% |
| Bathing/showering | 91% | 94% | 91% | 80% |
| Making hot drink/snack | 76% | 86% | 76% | 67% |
| Preparing hot meal | 98% | 96% | 97% | 93% |
| Number of weeks alive | 45.40 | 44.92 | 44.64 | 47.52 |
| **Resources per week** | | | | |
| Net cost to SSD | £37.82 | £33.28 | £38.97 | £28.49 |
| Hours home help | 3.69 | 1.52 | 3.68 | 1.54 |
| Cost of helpers | £16.35 | - | £16.66 | - |
| Days in day care | 0.21 | 0.18 | 0.26 | 0.18 |
| Days in LA home | 0.20 | 2.31 | 0.26 | 1.84 |
| HH as % of SSD cost | 20% | 26% | 20% | 27% |
| Scheme as % of SSD cost | 41% | - | 40% | - |
| Cost to NHS @ 5% discount | £46.99 | £26.60 | £38.66 | £17.83 |
| Visits by community nurse | 1.92 | 0.61 | 1.53 | 0.41 |
| Days as hospital in-patient | 0.93 | 0.62 | 0.75 | 0.42 |

This group at high risk of falling, like those with mobility problems, received a similar mixture of care manager activities as the average overall, as shown in Table 5.1.

*Incontinence*

On referral to the scheme incontinence of urine was identified for 24 per cent of the older people and incontinence of faeces for 13 per cent. This will tend, if anything, to be an underestimate in view of the embarrassment of older people initially to disclose such difficulties, or their acceptance of the idea that it is an inevitable feature of old age (Brocklehurst, 1978). Careful assessment on occasions led to the need to persuade a reluctant older person to be referred to medical services. Some inappropriate use of drugs such as diuretics was discovered where proper dosage or different times of administration of tablets, under the guidance of helpers, substantially resolved the problem. For older people with severe mobility problems or who were bedfast, a regular rota of visits from helpers and other carers was devised to help the older person use the toilet, thereby preventing incontinence, to empty catheters and to change pads. Such rotas were usually devised in conjunction with community nurses who were involved in advising and training helpers in techniques of managing incontinence. On a number of occasions, successful coping strategies could be seen to have had a direct impact on morale by restoring dignity and self-respect. It became possible to make further progress towards increasing a person's level of social contacts since they were no longer so afraid of experiencing the indignity of an 'accident'.

The complexity of managing incontinence at home is illustrated by Mrs S.:

Mrs S. was a very frail lady who had a number of strokes several years previously and suffered from Parkinson's disease. Her mobility was very limited. She needed help getting up and going to bed, washing, dressing, rising from a chair and with toileting. She had been living with a daughter who had more or less done everything for her. She was referred to the scheme by her general practitioner when her daughter suddenly died. She was adamant that she would not go into residential or nursing home care.

The night nursing service had provided a night sitter and the family felt that she couldn't be left overnight at all, or indeed for any length of time, as Mrs S. was very anxious about being alone. The continence adviser, district nurses and her two daughters were involved in discussions with the care manager about how to cope with Mrs S.'s need for help in getting to the toilet. Whilst care scheme staff got her to use the commode when they were there, there was no guarantee that this was when she needed the toilet, especially as she was taking diuretics. Mrs S. needed special incontinence pads, requiring guidance from the continence adviser. The aim was to leave Mrs S. on her own a little longer between each visit, to give her confidence without undermining her independence. This was achieved with a rota, which included family members, and private carers who stayed overnight, home help and care scheme helpers. Once the continence problem was under control Mrs S. could be left for longer periods until she achieved a degree of independence and was not totally dependent on someone being with her most of the time. Mrs S. also began to attend a lunch club, which was a great achievement since she had been housebound for some ten years.

Table 5.4 compares the characteristics of those who suffered from incontinence with the group as a whole. Those who were frequently incontinent of urine or faeces accounted for some 29 per cent of the care scheme group. They were more likely than average to be immobile or at frequent risk of falling and needed more help with activities of daily living such as dressings, toileting and bathing. These findings are similar to those of Challis and Davies (1986) in the

**Table 5.4**

*Comparison of those with incontinence problems with all*

| | Incontinence problem cases | | All cases | |
|---|---|---|---|---|
| | Care scheme | Comparison group | Care scheme | Comparison group |
| *Descriptive material* | | | | |
| Number of cases | 29 | 23 | 101 | 144 |
| Average age (years) | 81 | 81 | 81 | 80 |
| *Gender* | | | | |
| Male | 17% | 22% | 13% | 16% |
| Female | 83% | 78% | 87% | 84% |
| *Living group* | | | | |
| Alone | 79% | 52% | 75% | 69% |
| With spouse | 14% | 9% | 13% | 9% |
| Other | 7% | 39% | 12% | 22% |
| Presence of informal carer | 76% | 87% | 71% | 72% |
| *Outcomes* | | | | |
| At home | 55% | 44% | 62% | 46% |
| Local authority home | 3% | 17% | 2% | 29% |
| Private residential/nursing home | 0% | 0% | 0% | 2% |
| Long-term hospital care | 14% | 17% | 9% | 4% |
| Died | 28% | 22% | 26% | 18% |
| Moved away | 0% | 0% | 1% | 1% |
| *Problem prevalence* | | | | |
| Immobility | 48% | 78% | 44% | 36% |
| Incontinence (frequent) | 100% | 100% | 29% | 16% |
| Cognitive impairment (moderate or severe) | 41% | 43% | 31% | 30% |
| Instability (frequent falling risk) | 62% | 61% | 56% | 35% |
| Informal carer stress | 45% | 59% | 48% | 47% |
| Breathlessness | 66% | 48% | 57% | 51% |
| Giddiness | 55% | 52% | 64% | 55% |
| Eyesight | 83% | 56% | 75% | 65% |
| Hearing | 55% | 65% | 55% | 48% |
| Frequent loneliness | 48% | 62% | 57% | 61% |
| Depression (moderate or severe) | 45% | 52% | 55% | 56% |
| Anxiety (moderate or severe) | 41% | 52% | 58% | 56% |
| ADL index (0-6) | 4.2 | 4.8 | 3.4 | 2.5 |

**Table 5.4 (continued)**

| | Incontinence problem cases | | All cases | |
| --- | --- | --- | --- | --- |
| | Care scheme | Comparison group | Care scheme | Comparison group |
| *Needing help with activities of daily living* | | | | |
| Dressing | 79% | 78% | 60% | 36% |
| Getting to/using toilet | 90% | 91% | 63% | 41% |
| Feeding self (mechanical) | 10% | 10% | 13% | 12% |
| Bathing/showering | 97% | 100% | 91% | 80% |
| Making hot drink/snack | 83% | 91% | 76% | 67% |
| Preparing hot meal | 100% | 100% | 97% | 93% |
| Number of weeks alive | 42.60 | 45.52 | 44.64 | 47.52 |
| *Resources per week* | | | | |
| Net cost to SSD | £39.71 | £22.57 | £38.97 | £28.49 |
| Hours home help | 3.20 | 1.52 | 3.68 | 1.54 |
| Cost of helpers | £18.01 | - | £16.66 | - |
| Days in day care | 0.34 | 0.04 | 0.26 | 0.18 |
| Days in LA home | 0.33 | 1.43 | 0.26 | 1.84 |
| HH as % of SSD cost | 18% | 31% | 20% | 27% |
| Scheme as % of SSD cost | 40% | - | 40% | - |
| Cost to NHS @ 5% discount | £49.26 | £34.27 | £38.66 | £17.83 |
| Visits by community nurse | 1.07 | 0.55 | 1.53 | 0.41 |
| Days as hospital in-patient | 1.16 | 0.95 | 0.75 | 0.42 |

Kent scheme. Although these older people were, as expected, more likely to suffer from cognitive impairment, they appeared less frequently depressed or anxious. A higher proportion than average had a carer, as many of this group would not still be able to remain at home without this informal help. Slightly less than average were still at home a year later, while more were in long-term local authority or hospital care. This probably indicated that nursing input as part of the team would be required to support such older people, as was effected in the primary health care scheme, which is described in Chapter 9.

Weekly costs to the social services department of people suffering from incontinence were little more than average. However, costs to the National Health Service were markedly higher, mainly as a result of a greater number of days having been spent in hospital care.

The case review information in Table 5.1 indicates that more care manager activity was spent in advocacy and mobilising resources. This reflects again the need for nursing care inputs and the care managers' activity in liaising with the continence advisor.

*Intellectual impairment*

The management of dementia is perhaps the most demanding problem facing any community service. At first assessment, 31 per cent of the older people were identified as moderately or severely confused. In the original Kent scheme (Challis and Davies, 1986) the success of a more flexible approach with such cases was noted, and in Gateshead this was developed further.

In order to gain a clear picture of the extent of the problem, assessment for this group of elderly people took longer than average and needed to use a variety of different strategies. For example, people who were known to the older person and had already gained their trust were often recruited as helpers. The care manager would work through such a familiar face until able to gain trust and acceptance themselves. This has been described as the use of a wide range of strategies in 'gaining entrée' (Challis and Davies, 1986). One elderly woman consistently mistook her care manager for her granddaughter. This perception was not challenged since it permitted effective access to the lady and the acceptance of necessary help. In trying to understand the extent of the problem for an individual, one important element which was evident early on was the extent to which isolation, understimulation or sensory deprivation could magnify the impact of the condition. This secondary decline and loss of skills has been described elsewhere as 'process risk' (Challis and Davies, 1986). In the initial stages it was often necessary to tease out and eliminate possible contributory factors which could magnify the effect of mental impairment, such as undetected acute illnesses, urinary and chest infections or the effect of inappropriate administration of drugs. This required the immediate involvement of a specialist clinician.

Assessment often involved identifying cues which were relevant to the older person in order to preserve their remaining skills and build on these with appropriate forms of care (Berman and Rappaport, 1984). This could often involve examining the performance of specific tasks, as Mace and Rabins (1981) indicate, to determine the extent to which they could still do the task completely, safely and without becoming upset. For example, one elderly woman retained an approximate idea of the time of day from simply watching school children go past her window. Once this became apparent, the care manager had to devise strategies to help her cope with the effects of changing the clock and lighter evenings. The pace at which assessment, care planning and services could proceed was often slow and controlled so as to avoid overburdening the older person's remaining mental abilities. It was necessary to set care tasks and the objectives of support at a realistic level. Often an early gain, simply through the effect of stimulation, was observed and it was important to ensure that helpers were not disappointed at the subsequent setting of realistic, limited objectives. Identifying significant environmental factors could also influence care. Minimising risks from appliances such as cookers and gas fires could be achieved by changing the fuel supply and providing alternative means of heating. This could involve having the gas supply switched on only while others were in the house. Boiling a kettle dry could sometimes be avoided by supplying an automatic electric one, although perseverance and, indeed, further kettles could sometimes be required to teach the person not to put it on the cooker. Tackling these hazards was described in the Kent scheme as dealing with 'event risk' (Challis and Davies, 1986), associated with the loss of coping skills to the point where normal sequential acts of daily living are not completed in their entirety, such as turning on gas taps and failing to light them, thereby creating a danger both for the older person and their immediate environment.

The way in which help was offered in the approach of both the care manager and the helpers appeared to be crucial to effective outcomes. Often a pattern of one-to-one communication had to be resurrected as older people had often been talked over on the assumption that they were unable to understand. The use of simple reality orientation techniques could sometimes be useful, such as reminding people of the time of day, the meal being consumed and their location (Berman and Rappaport, 1984). In the case of one older woman who had moved into sheltered housing a large notice with her name and address was placed on the inside of her front door which appeared to give her effective cues. The care managers tried to ensure that these principles were part of the minutiae of the interactions between the older person and the helpers. Thus, instead of leaving the room to undertake a domestic task and later reappearing and confusing the older person, helpers were trained to respond by explaining that they were going to make tea and to ask the person if they wanted to come as well. Again, rather than disappearing upstairs to make the bed and reappearing later they would suggest that the older person assisted them in making the bed. The aim was wherever possible to keep the helper visible, involve the older person and provide a commentary about what was being done and why. Most importantly, such approaches needed to go hand in hand with work to build up a structured day. This has been described as 'patterning care' (Challis and Davies, 1986), a pattern of care based on the positive elements, abilities and routines of the person. It was vitally important to identify and preserve retained skills and behaviour patterns, even if this could take more time to achieve care objectives. One example was a woman who moved to sheltered housing and began to wander at night. It was discovered that her previous pattern had been to put rollers in her hair before undertaking the other tasks of retiring, such as washing and putting on her night-clothes. Therefore, a helper was enlisted to assist her with these tasks. By re-establishing this long-held routine she would then remain in bed until a helper called in the morning to take out the rollers. Another woman, also having moved into sheltered housing, was found to have had a habit at bedtime of changing her calendar to the next day, winding her clock and of folding two handkerchiefs in bed. In re-establishing this routine it was possible to ensure that she took her medication as part of the activity. Thus, the aim was to re-establish life patterns rather than impose an unfamiliar external routine, which is often inevitable using existing services. This required the care manager to identify what skills remained, and what was meaningful to the older person and to build on that identified routine.

On other occasions a structure of activities provided when the person was liable to become restless and wander, such as at bedtimes, could be sufficient to bridge the period of restlessness and make it possible to settle the person in bed. While attending day hospital it was discovered that one woman greatly enjoyed knitting dishcloths. A pattern was established that on retiring the helper would provide her with wool to knit a dishcloth to have ready for her in the morning. It was important to provide her with only sufficient wool for the one dishcloth otherwise she would continue regardless. Nonetheless, after this activity she was sufficiently tired to be able to pass the night without disturbing her neighbours. By providing a greater degree of structure, a number of people with confusional states were successfully introduced into day care groups where the use of recall and reminiscence revealed considerable valuable background information and provided clues as how to match the person's needs with help in a more acceptable fashion.

It appeared that for some cognitively impaired older people, care at home could be successful because it was organised around the individual in their own home, worked with what was familiar, and was sensitive to and did not disrupt any functional daily patterns which the person may have had. Another important aspect of managing older people suffering from dementia involved trying to relieve the stresses and strains facing carers.

Table 5.5 compares those with cognitive impairment with the group as a whole. These made up almost one third of the group, and all except two were female. Although a lower than average proportion were living with a spouse and more were living alone, a greater proportion had a carer than average. Moreover, an important part of the support provided in such cases was in offering help and relief to those providing informal care.

Incontinence was more common in this group, as would be expected (Challis and Davies, 1986), occurring in 39 per cent of cases. However, fewer than half the cases, 45 per cent, were at risk of falling. Nevertheless, paradoxically this could often put them at greater risk in other respects, through wandering and placing themselves at risk. Their physical health was generally above average, and the prevalence of breathlessness was much smaller than the care scheme group as a whole. Despite their better physical health, they needed similar or higher levels of assistance with activities of daily living. In addition, their carers experienced higher levels of stress than carers as a whole. There also appeared to be lower levels of depression and anxiety. Interestingly, in view of the increased risk of institutional care for individuals with cognitive impairment, evident in the comparison group, no such effect could be discerned for those receiving the care scheme. This suggests that the scheme was able considerably to reduce the risk of institutional care for these cases.

**Table 5.5**
*Comparison of those with cognitive impairment with all*

| | Cognitively impaired cases | | All cases | |
|---|---|---|---|---|
| | Care scheme | Comparison group | Care scheme | Comparison group |
| **Descriptive material** | | | | |
| Number of cases | 31 | 43 | 101 | 144 |
| Average age (years) | 83 | 81 | 81 | 80 |
| **Gender** | | | | |
| Male | 7% | 9% | 13% | 16% |
| Female | 93% | 91% | 87% | 84% |
| **Living group** | | | | |
| Alone | 84% | 67% | 75% | 69% |
| With spouse | 3% | 5% | 13% | 9% |
| Other | 13% | 28% | 12% | 22% |
| Presence of informal carer | 90% | 81% | 71% | 72% |
| **Outcomes** | | | | |
| At home | 61% | 33% | 62% | 46% |
| Local authority home | 3% | 32% | 2% | 29% |
| Private residential/nursing home | 0% | 0% | 0% | 2% |
| Long-term hospital care | 13% | 12% | 9% | 4% |
| Died | 23% | 23% | 26% | 18% |
| Moved away | 0% | 0% | 1% | 1% |
| **Problem prevalence** | | | | |
| Immobility | 42% | 35% | 44% | 36% |
| Incontinence (frequent) | 39% | 24% | 29% | 16% |
| Cognitive impairment (moderate or severe) | 100% | 100% | 31% | 30% |
| Instability (frequent falling risk) | 45% | 19% | 56% | 35% |
| Informal carer stress | 60% | 63% | 48% | 47% |
| Breathlessness | 29% | 42% | 57% | 51% |
| Giddiness | 58% | 58% | 64% | 55% |
| Eyesight | 73% | 54% | 75% | 65% |
| Hearing | 65% | 40% | 55% | 48% |
| Frequent loneliness | 53% | 64% | 57% | 61% |
| Depression (moderate or severe) | 39% | 58% | 55% | 56% |
| Anxiety (moderate or severe) | 48% | 58% | 58% | 56% |
| ADL index (0-6) | 3.5 | 2.6 | 3.4 | 2.5 |

**Table 5.5 (continued)**

|  | Cognitively impaired cases | | All cases | |
|  | Care scheme | Comparison group | Care scheme | Comparison group |
|---|---|---|---|---|
| *Needing help with activities of daily living* | | | | |
| Dressing | 71% | 44% | 60% | 36% |
| Getting to/using toilet | 64% | 42% | 63% | 41% |
| Feeding self (mechanical) | 3% | 12% | 13% | 12% |
| Bathing/showering | 90% | 79% | 91% | 80% |
| Making hot drink/snack | 94% | 84% | 76% | 67% |
| Preparing hot meal | 100% | 100% | 97% | 93% |
| Number of weeks alive | 43.36 | 45.40 | 44.64 | 47.52 |
| *Resources per week* | | | | |
| Net cost to SSD | £40.30 | £31.76 | £38.97 | £28.49 |
| Hours home help | 3.08 | 0.80 | 3.68 | 1.54 |
| Cost of helpers | £18.05 | - | £16.66 | - |
| Days in day care | 0.53 | 0.004 | 0.26 | 0.18 |
| Days in LA home | 0.28 | 2.32 | 0.26 | 1.84 |
| HH as % of SSD cost | 17% | 16% | 20% | 27% |
| Scheme as % of SSD cost | 41% | - | 40% | - |
| Cost to NHS @ 5% discount | £41.13 | £24.82 | £38.66 | £17.83 |
| Visits by community nurse | 1.34 | 0.56 | 1.53 | 0.41 |
| Days as hospital in-patient | 0.89 | 0.68 | 0.75 | 0.42 |

Social services weekly costs (£40.30) were slightly above the mean of £38.97 and one component of this, day care, was twice as frequently used. This provided some of the extra supervision necessary whilst allowing relief to carers. As in the Kent scheme, these older people in Gateshead received more support from helpers but less from the home help service (Challis and Davies, 1986), suggesting the need for more individualised and idiosyncratic forms of care.

From the case review information in Table 5.1 it can be seen that, unsurprisingly, the provision of information and advice and facilitating problem solving were less frequent for the cognitively impaired than average. However, as would be expectedly the care manager more frequently provided support to carers.

## Depressed mood

Depressed mood was evident for about 57 per cent of the older people. Such cases often receive services rather than a response to the mood state, which may often be presented in somatic form (Goldberg and Huxley, 1980; Challis

and Davies, 1986). Care managers appeared to be able to respond more effectively to the more situationally-determined mood states, often associated with
the range of losses experienced by older people, such as the loss of partner,
function and home. For such cases support from helpers to tackle isolation and
loneliness, providing the opportunity for social interaction sometimes met
with success. However, the more severe and chronic conditions were less amenable to social support, and tended to be a source of strain for helpers working
with them. Care at home of such individuals has been shown to be more likely
to break down both in another care management scheme (Challis et al., 1995)
and in a home care service (Lindesay and Murphy, 1989). Interestingly, links
with a specialist mental health service could well have improved the prognosis
of care for such cases (Bannerjee et al., 1996). An example is Mrs L., who was
unable to be maintained by the scheme in her own home and had to enter
long-term care:

> Mrs L. was described as chronically depressed, and proved unresponsive
> to all interventions. Her housing was poor in terms of situation, decor
> and furnishings. She smoked the whole time; this was all she wanted to
> do. She would not feed herself, walk from her chair or do anything in the
> house. She was uninterested in any social stimulation and had no con-
> versation. The helpers found her very hard work and unrewarding to
> care for, and felt they were getting nowhere. The only positive aspect was
> that the care manager did manage to form a relationship with her and
> when it became clear that the only option was long-term care, the care
> manager was able to talk through this with her. The care manager accom-
> panied her to visit the home and followed this up with later visits. Al-
> though the scheme was unable to maintain her in her own home, her
> transition to long-term care was made easier.

Table 5.6 compares those elderly people who suffered symptoms of depression with the group as a whole. Those who were rated as having moderate to
severe depressed mood were identified for this comparison. Of these, 80 per
cent suffered considerable anxiety, similar to the Kent study (Challis and
Davies, 1986). They were also slightly younger and fewer had a carer. As a consequence, a high proportion felt lonely for most of the time, compared with
those older people receiving the care scheme as a whole, again reflecting the
findings of Challis and Davies (1986). Risk of falling, giddiness and poor eyesight were more frequently found in this group, possibly reflecting an association with poor physical health.

Whereas in the comparison group a larger proportion entered institutional
care, those receiving the scheme were more likely to remain at home. Social
services department costs for care scheme cases were slightly higher. However,
costs to the National Health Service for the depressed group receiving the care
scheme were considerably higher than for the comparison group. This

**Table 5.6**
*Comparison of those with depression with all*

|  | Depressed cases | | All cases | |
|---|---|---|---|---|
|  | Care scheme | Comparison group | Care scheme | Comparison group |
| *Descriptive material* | | | | |
| Number of cases | 56 | 81 | 101 | 144 |
| Average age (years) | 79 | 79 | 81 | 80 |
| *Gender* | | | | |
| Male | 14% | 17% | 13% | 16% |
| Female | 86% | 83% | 87% | 84% |
| *Living group* | | | | |
| Alone | 73% | 74% | 75% | 69% |
| With spouse | 16% | 7% | 13% | 9% |
| Other | 11% | 19% | 12% | 22% |
| Presence of informal carer | 61% | 73% | 71% | 72% |
| *Outcomes* | | | | |
| At home | 60% | 38% | 62% | 46% |
| Local authority home | 4% | 37% | 2% | 29% |
| Private residential/nursing home | 0% | 1% | 0% | 2% |
| Long-term hospital care | 11% | 3% | 9% | 4% |
| Died | 25% | 20% | 26% | 18% |
| Moved away | 0% | 1% | 1% | 1% |
| *Problem prevalence* | | | | |
| Immobility | 38% | 36% | 44% | 36% |
| Incontinence (frequent) | 23% | 15% | 29% | 16% |
| Cognitive impairment (moderate or severe) | 21% | 31% | 31% | 30% |
| Instability (frequent falling risk) | 64% | 38% | 56% | 35% |
| Informal carer stress | 45% | 59% | 48% | 47% |
| Breathlessness | 63% | 63% | 57% | 51% |
| Giddiness | 75% | 66% | 64% | 55% |
| Eyesight | 84% | 67% | 75% | 65% |
| Hearing | 54% | 45% | 55% | 48% |
| Frequent loneliness | 77% | 82% | 57% | 61% |
| Depression (moderate or severe) | 100% | 100% | 55% | 56% |
| Anxiety (moderate or severe) | 80% | 75% | 58% | 56% |
| ADL index (0-6) | 3.2 | 2.6 | 3.4 | 2.5 |

Table 5.6 (continued)

| | Depressed cases | | All cases | |
|---|---|---|---|---|
| | Care scheme | Comparison group | Care scheme | Comparison group |
| *Needing help with activities of daily living* | | | | |
| Dressing | 56% | 38% | 60% | 36% |
| Getting to/using toilet | 55% | 44% | 63% | 41% |
| Feeding self (mechanical) | 14% | 14% | 13% | 12% |
| Bathing/showering | 91% | 79% | 91% | 80% |
| Making hot drink/snack | 75% | 67% | 76% | 67% |
| Preparing hot meal | 94% | 94% | 97% | 93% |
| Number of weeks alive | 45.16 | 47.60 | 44.64 | 47.52 |
| *Resources per week* | | | | |
| Net cost to SSD | £38.54 | £34.63 | £38.97 | £28.49 |
| Hours home help | 3.69 | 1.67 | 3.68 | 1.54 |
| Cost of helpers | £15.24 | - | £16.66 | - |
| Days in day care | 0.22 | 0.27 | 0.26 | 0.18 |
| Days in LA home | 0.35 | 2.29 | 0.26 | 1.84 |
| HH as % of SSD cost | 20% | 27% | 20% | 27% |
| Scheme as % of SSD cost | 38% | - | 40% | - |
| Cost to NHS @ 5% discount | £44.42 | £16.52 | £38.66 | £17.83 |
| Visits by community nurse | 1.72 | 0.35 | 1.53 | 0.41 |
| Days as hospital in-patient | 0.84 | 0.41 | 0.75 | 0.42 |

followed from the greater proportion of time that they spent in hospital, perhaps associated with their high risk of falling.

The frequency of care manager activities and contacts with other agencies (Table 5.1) did not differ significantly from the averages for all older people.

*Informal carers*

Families have too often been left to cope unaided or offered services which are of little help to their main concerns, being predominantly geared to meeting very different needs (Charlesworth et al., 1984; Henwood and Wicks, 1984; SSI, 1987). Meeting the needs of carers was a substantial part of the care scheme, as about two-thirds of the older people who received the scheme had carers. Of those, 65 per cent were identified as 'stressed' using the criteria of Rutter et al. (1970). Thus, overall, carer stress was a problem for 49 per cent of older people supported by the scheme. Since existing services tend not to focus on the needs of families or may be less appropriate to their concerns, it was not uncommon that the care scheme was the only support available to assist carers. The help given was very varied; ranging from providing relief to people who lived with the older person, to assisting carers who lived nearby and called frequently. On some occasions it was necessary to deal with considerable conflict in a care network, arising from misperceptions between the older person and carer, and attempting to resolve problems of hidden stress, guilt and difficulties in relationships. On other occasions work involved shifting the balance of demands within family groups to avoid polarisation of care on one individual (Ratna and Davis, 1984).

Sometimes it was clear that the contribution of carers was inappropriate, as for instance when they might keep the older person in bed all the time or where the carer might be unable to offer intimate care of the kind required. Consequently, it was necessary to identify what tasks the carer was willing and able to undertake so that an acceptable level of shared input could be achieved with the aim of maintaining a relationship of value to the older person while improving their quality of care. On some occasions where an excessive burden was experienced by the carer carrying almost sole responsibility, the helpers had to be introduced gradually until such time as trust in the quality of alternative care was established. The kind of help offered could vary from providing types of support not normally available, to undertaking tasks at times when other services did not. This could perhaps involve offering a sitting service so that carers could have time to undertake activities in their personal lives, or 'doubling up' whereby a helper could assist a carer with helping the older person in and out of bed or with other activities. On occasions in working with carers a great deal of effort had to be made to unravel the original support network and encourage friends and relatives to withdraw. For example, an older woman suffering from anxiety, depression and increasing physical frailty had a daughter who was the sole carer. The demands of this caused severe stress for the daughter and was causing problems in her marriage. Nonetheless, she felt duty-bound every day to go back and forth to her mother and, despite the effects on her own health and family, could not envisage any alternative to her own care. The care manager had to work at gradually substituting the daughter's input, while making this acceptable to the woman. After a period of time the daughter's involvement was that of social visiting rather than hands-on caring. Such cases emphasise very clearly the 'direct' work element, such as counselling, in the scheme.

At times confusion and misunderstanding can occur in the relationship between social services departments and carers, due to the conflicting role models. It can sometimes be unclear whether the carer is an additional resource, a service user in their own right or a co-worker (Twigg, 1989). This condition was less likely to occur in the care scheme, where older people with carers received markedly higher levels of support, a more careful assessment and an involvement in care planning to identify which roles the carer was willing and able to undertake.

Table 5.7 compares the characteristics of those whose carer exhibited signs and symptoms of stress and strain with those of the group as a whole. Those whose carer had a Malaise score of 5 and over were selected for this category

**Table 5.7**
*Comparison of those with a stressed informal carer with all*

| | Stressed carer cases | | All cases | |
| | Care scheme | Comparison group | Care scheme | Comparison group |
|---|---|---|---|---|
| *Descriptive material* | | | | |
| Number of cases | 48 | 66 | 101 | 144 |
| Average age (years) | 80 | 80 | 81 | 80 |
| *Gender* | | | | |
| Male | 8% | 17% | 13% | 16% |
| Female | 92% | 83% | 87% | 84% |
| *Living group* | | | | |
| Alone | 71% | 60% | 75% | 69% |
| With spouse | 13% | 11% | 13% | 9% |
| Other | 16% | 29% | 12% | 22% |
| Presence of informal carer | 100% | 100% | 71% | 72% |
| *Outcomes* | | | | |
| At home | 54% | 41% | 62% | 46% |
| Local authority home | 4% | 29% | 2% | 29% |
| Private residential/nursing home | 0% | 0% | 0% | 2% |
| Long-term hospital care | 13% | 4% | 9% | 4% |
| Died | 27% | 26% | 26% | 18% |
| Moved away | 2% | 0% | 1% | 1% |
| *Problem prevalence* | | | | |
| Immobility | 44% | 38% | 44% | 36% |
| Incontinence (frequent) | 27% | 20% | 29% | 16% |
| Cognitive impairment (moderate or severe) | 38% | 41% | 31% | 30% |
| Instability (frequent falling risk) | 60% | 35% | 56% | 35% |
| Informal carer stress | 100% | 100% | 48% | 47% |
| Breathlessness | 50% | 58% | 57% | 51% |
| Giddiness | 67% | 59% | 64% | 55% |
| Eyesight | 79% | 68% | 75% | 65% |
| Hearing | 48% | 39% | 55% | 48% |
| Frequent loneliness | 55% | 53% | 57% | 61% |
| Depression (moderate or severe) | 52% | 71% | 55% | 56% |
| Anxiety (moderate or severe) | 65% | 68% | 58% | 56% |
| ADL index (0-6) | 3.5 | 2.8 | 3.4 | 2.5 |

**Table 5.7 (continued)**

|  | Stressed carer cases | | All cases | |
|  | Care scheme | Comparison group | Care scheme | Comparison group |
|---|---|---|---|---|
| *Needing help with activities of daily living* | | | | |
| Dressing | 73% | 41% | 60% | 36% |
| Getting to/using toilet | 33% | 44% | 63% | 41% |
| Feeding self (mechanical) | 12% | 16% | 13% | 12% |
| Bathing/showering | 92% | 86% | 91% | 80% |
| Making hot drink/snack | 80% | 76% | 76% | 67% |
| Preparing hot meal | 96% | 96% | 97% | 93% |
| Number of weeks alive | 43.08 | 44.56 | 44.64 | 47.52 |
| *Resources per week* | | | | |
| Net cost to SSD | £37.65 | £30.16 | £38.97 | £28.49 |
| Hours home help | 2.98 | 1.17 | 3.68 | 1.54 |
| Cost of helpers | £14.83 | - | £16.66 | - |
| Days in day care | 0.35 | 0.24 | 0.26 | 0.18 |
| Days in LA home | 0.36 | 2.01 | 0.26 | 1.84 |
| HH as % of SSD cost | 17% | 21% | 20% | 27% |
| Scheme as % of SSD cost | 36% | - | 40% | - |
| Cost to NHS @ 5% discount | £48.09 | £25.47 | £38.66 | £17.83 |
| Visits by community nurse | 1.23 | 0.36 | 1.53 | 0.41 |
| Days as hospital in-patient | 0.92 | 0.59 | 0.75 | 0.42 |

(Rutter et al., 1970). Almost half of all older people receiving the scheme, 48 out of 101, had a stressed carer.

Two particular problem areas appeared to be associated with carer stress, more than for the group as a whole. These were presence of cognitive impairment and anxiety in the older person. Fifty-four per cent were still at home a year later compared with the average of 62 per cent. More of these older people entered long-term hospital care. It is possible that the support provided by the carer was more likely to break down over a prolonged period, even with the support of the care scheme. However, the rate of breakdown of care was greater for the comparison group.

The average weekly cost to the National Health Service of £48.09 was larger than the average of £38.66, due to the greater time spent in hospital. However, inner city average weekly national health service costs were less than half those in the outer city, owing to fewer community nursing visits and less time having been spent as a hospital in-patient. To compensate for this, social services department costs in the inner city were much higher, due to greater helper costs, more day care and more local authority residential care being deployed by the care manager.

The case review material in Table 5.1 shows that the care managers spent more time giving support to these stressed carers, compared with the group as a whole. Nevertheless, it is perhaps surprising that this figure was not still higher.

### The effect of presence of a carer and living group on location at one year

This section examines the impact of different types of need category and the presence or absence of a carer upon the probability of remaining at home. There was relatively little variation in the percentage of care scheme cases entering permanent institutional care according to the type of need category. This ranged from 19 per cent for cases at frequent risk of falling to 24 per cent for those who were frequently incontinent.

For older people with no carer, who mostly lived alone, admissions to institutional care were the exception (4 per cent). Most cases with a carer lived alone and of these only 14 per cent entered institutional care. The effect of different needs upon admission rates differed according to carer support. A lower proportion of those with cognitive impairment, living alone and without a carer remained at home than those with a carer. Conversely, the impact of depression and incontinence was in the other direction.

Comparisons of the relative impact of the scheme were made by examining the effect of levels of carer support and need group upon matched experimental and comparison cases. The largest reduction in the admission rate (subtracting comparison group admissions from experimental ones) was achieved for depressed cases (38 per cent) followed by those who were confused or at risk of falling (35 per cent) and carer stress (31 per cent). From examining the effect of different levels of carer input, it was clear that cases living alone without a carer experienced the greatest reduction in admission (54 per cent). The greatest reduction in admission rate was achieved for those at risk of falling (58 per cent) followed by those suffering incontinence (50 per cent). Regarding those with cognitive impairment, of those living alone the reduction in admissions was lower (27 per cent) than for those living alone with a non-resident carer (39 per cent).

Older people's circumstances clearly influenced outcome, patterns of response and, as will be evident later, costs. Certainly, in the analysis of work with older people with cognitive impairment it was the pattern of response that proved to be the important factor. Even when trends of costliness or probability of entry to long-term care between the experimental and comparison groups were not dissimilar, the support of the care scheme appeared to attenuate these effects.

# 6 Outcomes for Older People

Earlier chapters have examined the pattern and type of care services offered by the care scheme. This chapter considers the outcomes of care for older people who received the care scheme service, compared with the outcomes for those receiving standard services.

### Characteristics of the older people

During the period of monitoring the scheme, 101 older people were referred and accepted as appropriate. They are described in Table 6.1. It can be seen that they constitute a frail group with an average age of 81 and predominantly female. Over two-thirds had a carer, of whom two-thirds were seen as under stress. Incontinence and confusion were problems affecting one-third of cases, while immobility and risk of falling affected a higher proportion. Most required help with key activities of daily living and all needed help with household chores. In terms of targeting the scheme therefore, they were a group with considerable needs in a variety of areas. With regard to outcomes, the consequences of not meeting need effectively for such a vulnerable group would be likely to impact upon the probability of residential placement, quality of life and quality of care of both the older people and their carers.

### Outcomes of care

As described in Chapter 2, older people receiving the care scheme were compared with a similar matched group of older people receiving the usual range of services. This section considers the findings from comparing these two matched groups of older people. First, an examination is made of the outcome

 UNIVERSITY OF WINCHESTER LIBRARY

**Table 6.1**
*Characteristics of the older people*[a]

| | |
|---|---|
| Mean age | 81 |
| *Gender* | |
| Male | 13% |
| Female | 87% |
| *Living group* | |
| Alone | 75% |
| Spouse | 13% |
| Family | 11% |
| Other | 1% |
| *Incontinence* | |
| Urine | 24% |
| Faeces | 13% |
| High risk of falling | 56% |
| Presence of confusional state | 31% |
| *Activities of daily living requiring assistance* | |
| Moving indoors on level | 39% |
| Preparing meals | 97% |
| Making hot drinks | 76% |
| Dressing/undressing | 60% |
| Feeding self | 13% |
| Managing medication | 66% |
| Bathing | 91% |
| Shopping | 100% |
| Cleaning | 100% |
| Getting to/using toilet | 63% |
| Getting in/out of bed/chair | 44% |
| Has carer | 71% |
| Carer under stress | 65%[b] |

a Based on 101 cases.
b Of 72 carers.

of care in terms of the location of the older person at the end of a 12-month period, then attention is given to measures of quality of life and quality of care for older people over one year, and finally an examination is made of the factors associated with improvements in quality of care and quality of life over the same time period.

*Location at one year*

Maintenance of independence, defined as community tenure, has long been one of the objectives of intensive care management. Table 6.2 shows the

**Table 6.2**
*Location at one year*

| Location | Care scheme | | Comparison group | |
|---|---|---|---|---|
| | *Number* | *%* | *Number* | *%* |
| Own home | 57 | 63 | 32 | 36 |
| Local authority home | 1 | 1 | 33 | 37 |
| Private or voluntary home | 0 | 0 | 2 | 2 |
| Hospital care | 6 | 7 | 4 | 4 |
| Died | 25 | 28 | 18 | 20 |
| Moved away | 1 | 1 | 1 | 1 |
| Total | 90 | 100 | 90 | 100 |

Overall chi-squared test: $X^2 = 40.7$ (p < 0.001).

location, defined as the permanent place of residence at one year for the 90 matched pairs of older people. It can be seen that whereas 63 per cent of those who received the scheme remained in their own homes, only 36 per cent of the comparison group did so. Not dissimilar numbers of each group were in long-stay hospitals, although there was a very marked difference in the rate of admission to residential homes. Only one per cent of those receiving the scheme were in a residential home at the end of one year compared with 39 per cent receiving the usual range of services. These differences between the care scheme and comparison groups were significant ($X^2 = 40.7$; p < 0.001).

It is noticeable that these results are similar to the findings of the Kent scheme, where 69 per cent remained in their own homes after one year, compared with 34 per cent of the comparison group. However, an even lower percentage of people in Gateshead entered residential homes than in the Kent scheme: one per cent in Gateshead and 12 per cent in Kent (Challis and Davies, 1986). The Kent study found a difference in the death rate of the two groups, the care scheme group appearing to survive longer. This was not evident here and there was no significant difference in the death rates. Nor was there a significant difference in the average length of survival over the year, 44 weeks for those receiving the care scheme and 46.5 weeks for the comparison group out of a possible 52 weeks.

Indeed, despite the care taken to match cases there was a slightly higher degree of physical frailty in the care scheme group which could well be a partial explanation for the slightly higher, albeit not significantly so, death rate for this group. It was noteworthy that of those who died and received the care scheme, 80 per cent died in their own homes or in short-term hospital care rather than long-term institutional care. This was seen as desirable by both older people and their carers, and in the comparison group the comparable figure was only 61 per cent.

Over one year those receiving the care scheme remained in their own homes on average for 43 weeks compared with only 33 weeks for those receiving the usual range of services (p < 0.001). The scheme appears to have enabled older people to remain in their own homes for longer and, in most cases, avoid entry to long-stay care. The greater proportion of the comparison group who entered long-stay care reflects the findings of other studies; namely that the lack of appropriate services may result in unnecessary admission to long-stay care (Sinclair, 1990). This is a pragmatic operationalisation of the diffuse concept of 'choice', by reducing the difference between level of resources required for residential care and that usually offered as maximum domiciliary support. There are many reports of the ineffectiveness of standard service provision reflecting this resource gap. This appears to be due to several interlinked reasons. First, there is a shortage of resources. It has been suggested that when services are provided to very frail older people, this is often not at an adequate level (Levin et al., 1989; Sinclair, 1990; Allen et al., 1992). Second, service provision has been shown to be inflexible, and not responsive to the needs of the older person (Dexter and Harbert, 1983; Challis and Davies, 1986; Challis et al., 1995). Third, there is a lack of service integration (Audit Commission, 1986; Sinclair and Williams, 1990a,b; Challis et al., 1995).

*Factors associated with remaining at home*

As noted earlier, there were marked differences between the care scheme and comparison groups in their respective probabilities of an older person remaining at home, which was one of the key objectives of the scheme. Hence, an examination was made of the factors associated with remaining at home, separately for those receiving the scheme and the comparison group, so as to tease out the different factors involved. The method used was logistic regression analysis, which is a multi-variate technique designed to predict the probability of a binary outcome, in this case whether or not someone remained at home over a one-year period. The variables used in this analysis are shown in Box 6.1. Whilst those receiving the care scheme may have had more effective care, which may have enhanced their ability to remain at home, this analysis is concerned with questions of targeting and therefore resource variables have been omitted.

Table 6.3 shows the factors associated with remaining at home for those receiving the care scheme. Those who were more resistant to receiving help and those who appeared to have a passive attitude were less likely to remain at home. A similar effect appeared to be found in cost analyses in the Kent scheme (Challis and Davies, 1986). The presence of heart disease made it more likely that people would not remain at home, reflecting the influence of ill health on entry to care (Neill et al., 1988). Similarly, the presence of a stressed carer also reduced the likelihood of remaining at home (Levin et al., 1989, 1994), nonetheless, it must be remembered that markedly more of those

**Box 6.1**
*Variables used in predicting outcomes*

| DOMAIN/VARIABLE | VARIABLE FORM |
|---|---|
| **Health and dependency** | |
| Need for extra help with personal and household care | Sum of standardised needs[a] |
| Arthritis | None, moderate, severe |
| Eyesight difficulties | None, moderate, severe |
| Hearing difficulties | None, moderate, severe |
| Giddiness | None, moderate, severe |
| Breathlessness | None, moderate, severe |
| Heart problems | None, moderate, severe |
| Risk of falling | None, moderate, severe |
| Incontinence of urine | None, occasional, frequent |
| Incontinence of faeces | None, occasional, frequent |
| Dependency group 2 — short interval need | Presence or absence |
| Dependency group 3 — critical interval need | Presence or absence |
| Dependency group 4 — severe critical interval need | Presence or absence |
| Confusion/disorientation | Sum of responses to items concerning behaviour, appearance, memory; range 0-9 |
| Mental confusion | None, mild, moderate, severe |
| Depressed mood | None, mild, moderate, severe |
| PGC morale scale | Range 0-17 |
| Felt capacity to cope | Sum of responses to four questions concerning capacity to cope with different areas of daily living; range 4-16 |
| Loneliness | Sum of responses to two questions concerning felt loneliness and dissatisfaction; range 0-6 |
| Anxiety | None, mild, moderate, severe |
| General health problem index | Range 1-18 |
| Activities of daily living score | Range 0-6 |
| **Social support** | |
| All informal care | Social contact, score |
| Living with spouse | Presence or absence |
| Living with family | Presence or absence |
| Support from children | Number of weekly contacts |
| Support from relatives | Number of weekly contacts |
| Support from neighbours and friends | Number of weekly contacts |
| Support from informal carer | Presence or absence |
| Whether has confidant(e) | Presence or absence |
| **Personality and attitudes to help** | |
| Hostile–rejecting | Presence or absence |
| Independent — requires persuasion | Presence or absence |
| Passive–dependent | Presence or absence |
| Dependent–demanding | Presence or absence |

---

**Box 6.1 (continued)**

| DOMAIN/VARIABLE | VARIABLE FORM |
|---|---|
| **Other factors regarding older person** | |
| Age | Years |
| Gender | Male or female |
| Whether retired to area | Yes or no |
| Bereavement during past year | Yes or no |
| Whether living in inner city | Yes or no |
| Shortcomings in housing | Number of identified problems |
| **Initial effect on informal carer** | |
| Malaise score of stress symptoms | Range 0-24 |
| Practical problem score through caring | Range 0-8 |
| **Amount of resources provided** | |
| Residential care (local authority old people's home or private residential/ nursing home) | Days |
| Home help | Hours |
| Care scheme helpers' fees and expenses (proxy for time spent) | Pounds |
| Meals-on-wheels | Number |
| Day care | Days |
| Care manager time | Hours |
| Area team social worker time | Hours |
| Community nursing time | Hours |
| Hospital inpatient | Days |
| Geriatric/psychogeriatric day hospital | Days |
| Whether in long-term institutional care | Yes or no |

a Needs for extra help with (i) rising and retiring, (ii) personal care, (iii) daily housework, (iv) weekly housework, were standardised and then summed.

---

receiving the scheme remained at home, including those with carers. In general, studies of applications for local authority care have suggested that for about two-thirds, problems associated with carers make up one of the reasons for admission (Neill et al., 1988). Almost significant ($p = 0.09$) was the gender of the older person, where a female was more likely to remain at home. This reflects findings of other studies where men living alone may be more likely to apply for residential care than women in similar circumstances (Sinclair, 1990). In this study three-quarters of the older people were in fact living alone.

Table 6.4 shows the factors associated with remaining at home for the comparison group. These factors appear quite different and their explanatory power was lower (Lave's adj. $R^2 = 0.17$). Both the presence of confusional states and anxiety were associated with a lower probability of remaining at home. This reflects the findings of other studies on the problems of caring for

**Table 6.3**
*Predicting survival at home after one year for matched care scheme cases in terms of their initial characteristics*

| Variable | Coefficient | p value |
| --- | --- | --- |
| **Health and dependency** | | |
| Heart problems | -0.78 | <0.05 |
| **Personality and attitude to help** | | |
| Hostile–rejecting attitude | -2.27 | <0.05 |
| Passive–dependent attitude | -2.52 | <0.05 |
| **Other factors** | | |
| Gender: whether female | 1.43 | 0.09 |
| **Initial effect on informal carer** | | |
| Malaise score of stress symptoms | -0.10 | <0.05 |
| Constant | -0.86 | NS |

Percentage of correct predictions = 78
Lave's adjusted $R^2$ = 0.30
Number of cases = 90

**Table 6.4**
*Predicting survival at home after one year for matched comparison cases in terms of their initial characteristics*

| Variable | Coefficient | p value |
| --- | --- | --- |
| **Health and dependency** | | |
| Confusion/disorientation | -0.23 | 0.07 |
| Anxiety | -0.76 | 0.01 |
| **Social support** | | |
| Social contact scores | -0.04 | 0.09 |
| Constant | -0.24 | NS |

Percentage of correct predictions = 66
Lave's adjusted $R^2$ = 0.17
Number of cases = 90

those with cognitive impairment, and the particular difficulties of caring for those with confusion, at home (Sinclair, 1988; Levin et al., 1989, 1994). The level of social contact was also associated with likelihood of remaining at home; those with fewer contacts were less likely to remain at home. This factor may reflect the level of concern on the part of services and others to apparent risk. On the part of the older person it may reflect the findings of Allen et al. (1992) that a lack of social support, or an associated degree of loneliness, is a significant reason for admission to care homes.

Unsurprisingly, in both of these analyses it proved difficult to predict a phenomenon as complex and subject to multiple causes as survival at home. Nonetheless, the factors that entered the equations have apparent validity in that they are consistent with studies of why older people enter residential and nursing home care. Overall, the scheme was able to reduce the probability of entry to care, and although it appeared that the factors that precipitated this event remained those identified in earlier work, in practice their effect appears to have been attenuated.

### Quality of life and quality of care

Quality of life and quality of care outcomes were calculated by subtracting the initial value of a particular indicator when the older person was first interviewed from its value at follow-up one year later. The average change for those receiving the care scheme could then be compared with that for the comparison group. Those who had died or moved away were excluded from the comparison because of the absence of data at 12 months. This meant that even if matched groups had been used as a basis for investigation, the survivors who were analysed would no longer have been initially matched. It was therefore decided to start with unmatched groups as these allowed rather larger groups to be compared. As the measurement was of changes between two points in time, rather than level at follow-up, most of the effects that might be attributed to any mismatch were eliminated. Allowance was made for any effect of group mismatch on significance levels by testing the effects of initial matching variables as covariates in the analysis of variance, so as to ensure consistency in interpretation.

Some of the changes observed in quality of life or quality of care depended on whether the person was located at home or in institutional care after one year. Thus, whereas it might be expected that older people in institutional care would usually have their personal care and household needs satisfactorily catered for, this would not necessarily be the case for those remaining at home. Therefore, in order to gain insight into how institutional care could affect outcomes, the groups have also been sub-divided by whether after one year their permanent location was at home or in institutional care, as well as by whether they had received the care scheme. Comparisons were made between the groups using two-way analysis of variance, testing for both the effect of experimental/comparison group membership and the effect of location after one year.

*Quality of life* Table 6.5 shows the outcomes on a range of quality of life indicators for the older person, reflecting aspects of psychological well-being. As noted earlier, the analysis has examined not only whether experimental or comparison group membership determined the outcome but also the effects of whether or not a person entered residential or hospital care. Hence, for each

**Table 6.5**
*Social and emotional needs outcomes*

| Variable | | Mean | | Tests | |
|---|---|---|---|---|---|
| | | E | C | EvC | HvI |
| Depressed mood | Home: | -4.2 | -0.6 | <0.01 | <0.05 |
| | Inst.: | -2.8 | -3.7 | | |
| Loneliness | Home: | -1.2 | 0.1 | <0.001* | <0.01 |
| | Inst.: | 0.2 | -1.1 | | |
| Going out/social visits per week | Home: | 1.4 | -0.1 | <0.01 | <0.001 |
| | Inst.: | -1.0 | -1.9 | | |
| Morale | Home: | 2.1 | 0.6 | 0.08 | <0.01 |
| | Inst.: | 2.0 | 2.9 | | |
| Dissatisfaction with life development | Home: | -0.5 | 0.1 | <0.05 | <0.01 |
| | Inst.: | -0.6 | -0.7 | | |
| General dissatisfaction | Home: | -0.8 | -0.2 | 0.09 | 0.07 |
| | Inst.: | -0.8 | -0.9 | | |
| Felt capacity to cope | Home: | 4.9 | -0.1 | <0.001* | <0.001 |
| | Inst.: | 7.3 | 6.8 | | |
| Independence | Home: | 0.4 | -0.6 | 0.08 | ns |
| | Inst.: | -1.3 | -0.4 | | |

E = experimental group; C = comparison group; H = home; I = institution.
* = significant interaction effect.

indicator there are four scores: the mean change for those who received the care scheme or standard provision and remained in their own home, and the mean change for those who received the care scheme or standard provision and entered institutional care. The numbers in the care scheme group who entered institutional care were relatively few, but it was felt that this analysis would help to tease out further the factors that contributed to positive well-being.

For five of the indicators in Table 6.5, save the overall morale indicator, there was a significant positive advantage to those who received the care scheme. They were more likely to have improved in terms of depressed mood, loneliness, dissatisfaction with life (which is a component of morale), their felt capacity to cope and their level of social activity. There was also a significant positive effect for these subjective indicators — loneliness, depression and morale — associated with entry to institutional care, mainly due to the consequent improvement in the comparison group who entered homes. There were nearly significant positive effects for overall morale, independence or control over their own life, and a reduction in overall dissatisfaction. On the whole, the worst outcomes were observed for those comparison group cases who remained in their homes and received the existing range of domiciliary services. On the measure of loneliness it is noteworthy that the greatest improvement in the care scheme group was for those remaining in their own homes but for the comparison group improvement was greatest for those entering institutional care. However, on a measure of social activity, those receiving the scheme benefited most, and unsurprisingly those entering institutional care were least likely to go out and have social visits. The measure of the person's perception of their capacity to cope was improved both for those receiving the care scheme and for those entering institutional care. Only for those receiving existing services and remaining at home was there a decline in the older person's perception of their security. In terms of health-related quality of life, those receiving the care scheme experienced lower decline in activities of daily living, and it was noteworthy that experimental group cases who entered institutional care had experienced the greatest decline.

*Quality of care* Table 6.6 shows changes in assessments of need for additional help with a range of activities of daily living, the adequacy and quality of help, and need for additional services over the one year period. For the five measures of need, a minus sign indicates improvement, a reduction in the level of need. The measures of reliability, effectiveness and sufficiency of care are based upon older people's responses to the sum of specific questions about the help received across the four domains of rising and retiring; personal care; daily household care, such as meal provision; and weekly household care, such as laundry. The measures of adequacy are based upon the totals of the reliability, effectiveness and sufficiency of care within each of these four domains.

It can be seen that there is again a very consistent pattern for all the indicators in this table, similar to that shown in Table 6.5. Reductions of need are significantly greater for those receiving the scheme than for the comparison group with regard to getting up and going to bed, personal care, household care and number of services required. Entry to institutional care also appears to have benefited significantly both older people receiving the care scheme and those in the comparison group. However, remaining at home with existing services provided the worst outcome for the comparison group, particularly on indicators of personal care, daily household care and need for extra services, where this effect was highly significant. Similarly, on indicators of the older person's perception of the reliability, effectiveness and sufficiency of care received, those receiving the scheme appeared to have benefited significantly more than those receiving the usual range of services. Those entering institutional care also benefited significantly. Only those remaining at home and receiving the usual range of services appeared not to benefit, as can be seen from the significant interaction effect in this analysis. The indicators of adequacy of help present a similar picture. With regard to going out of the home, whereas those receiving the scheme were able to go out more frequently, others did not do so. Other potential problem areas were also affected by the

**Table 6.6**
*Care needs outcomes*

| Variable | | Mean | | Tests | |
|---|---|---|---|---|---|
| | | E | C | EvC | HvI |
| Need for help — a.m./p.m. | Home: | -2.2 | 0.4 | <0.001 | <0.001 |
| | Inst: | -2.6 | -1.6 | | |
| Need for help — personal care | Home: | -42.6 | 2.8 | <0.001* | <0.001 |
| | Inst.: | -33.0 | -23.4 | | |
| Need for help — daily household care | Home: | -16.2 | 0.5 | <0.001* | <0.001 |
| | Inst.: | -18.3 | -12.9 | | |
| Need for help — weekly household care | Home: | -5.9 | 0.8 | <0.001 | <0.001 |
| | Inst.: | -16.4 | -9.7 | | |
| Need for extra services | Home: | -6.2 | 0.1 | <0.001* | <0.001 |
| | Inst.: | -7.8 | -5.3 | | |
| Reliability of care | Home: | 5.0 | 0.2 | <0.001* | <0.001 |
| | Inst.: | 6.6 | 6.4 | | |
| Effectiveness of care | Home: | 3.4 | 0.0 | <0.001 | <0.001 |
| | Inst.: | 3.7 | 3.0 | | |
| Sufficiency of care | Home: | 7.1 | -0.1 | <0.001* | <0.001 |
| | Inst.: | 6.5 | 5.5 | | |
| Adequacy of help — a.m./p.m. | Home: | 3.3 | -0.1 | <0.001* | <0.001 |
| | Inst.: | 5.0 | 4.1 | | |
| Adequacy of help — personal care | Home: | 7.4 | -0.3 | <0.001* | <0.001 |
| | Inst.: | 6.1 | 5.5 | | |
| Adequacy of help — daily household care | Home: | 4.9 | 0.3 | <0.001* | <0.001 |
| | Inst.: | 6.2 | 5.4 | | |
| Adequacy of help — weekly household care | Home: | 2.4 | 0.3 | <0.001* | <0.001 |
| | Inst.: | 4.6 | 4.6 | | |
| | Home: | 1.4 | -0.1 | <0.01 | <0.001 |
| Frequency of getting out | Inst.: | -1.0 | -1.9 | | |

E = Experimental group; C = Comparison group; H = Home; I = Institution
* = Significant interaction effect

intervention of the scheme, indicated a reduction (p < 0.05) in problems associated with heating for those receiving the care scheme.

Thus, it would not be unreasonable to conclude from Tables 6.5 and 6.6 that of the four possible options, receiving the care scheme or standard services and entry to institutional care or remaining at home, that three out of four seemed to produce positive benefits from the point of view of the older person. The fourth however, did not. That fourth option was to receive the standard range of services and remain at home. For this highly dependent population the standard range of domiciliary services, despite the best efforts of those involved in providing them, are insufficient to meet the needs of the highly dependent elderly. This reflects the arguments of the Audit Commission (1986) and the findings of Levin et al. (1989) and Allen et al. (1992).

*Welfare gain — an alternative measure of output* The focus of the approach in measuring outcome has been to consider the changes in status between well-being at one point in time and at follow-up. The difference between these two points may be considered as the outcome of the experience of different modes of care. One aspect of outcome that such an approach does not address is the effect upon a person's well-being through time of states of well-being. Thus, for example, if a person were to experience a change in state just prior to their follow-up, they would be recorded as having the same outcome as a person who had enjoyed the same change in state for nine months. In order to make some allowance for this temporal effect on welfare the concept of 'welfare gain' was formulated. This was based upon the concept of 'Health Gain' (Cm 1523, 1992). In this, an attempt was made to take account of the gain experienced from different types of provision, care management or standard provision, by attempting to allow for the levels of well-being at intermediate stages of the evaluation year.

A full picture could of course only be obtained from knowledge of the level of well-being at all times during the period, which was not feasible. However, a simple approach was developed which rested on the clear evidence of difference between different types of setting in their impact upon outcomes. Earlier in the chapter the differences between the level of well-being for those at home and in institutional care for both experimental and comparison groups was noted. Some allowance was made for these fluctuations by assuming that the mean value of improvement in well-being for people who remained at home was representative of all periods spent at home for all individuals, while the corresponding value for people who moved into institutional care was representative of all periods spent in institutional care for all individuals, with experimental and comparison groups being considered separately. Welfare gain over the year was then estimated by weighting the improvement in outcome while at home by the average period spent at home and adding the improvement in outcome while in institutional care weighted by the average period spent in institutional care.

Using the same indicators as were used earlier in the chapter, it was found that by this method of calculating outcome the difference between experimental and comparison groups remained, with those receiving the care scheme exhibiting markedly higher welfare gain. This effect was particularly evident for the quality of care outcomes despite the gains for older people in the comparison group who entered residential care settings. The difference was attributable mainly to the poorest outcome being that of remaining at home and receiving the existing range of services.

### Factors influencing outcomes

The level of outcomes achieved for older people would be expected to depend on their initial characteristics and needs, and the quantity and quality of different types of resource consumed over the time period when outcomes were monitored. The nature and quality of the social services department itself and the teams providing support would also influence outcomes, though these would tend to affect all those receiving the care scheme to a similar degree, and the comparison group to a different degree. Furthermore, intermediate outcomes, such as whether or not the person was admitted to long-term institutional care, could also overall influence the outcomes.

Outcomes influenced by these types of factor were predicted by means of a production function (Knapp, 1984). The outcomes, which in this instance were the measures of quality of life or quality of care, were predicted by means of the non-resource inputs made up of characteristics of the older person and carer (quasi-inputs) and resource inputs expressed as the number of units of different types of resource consumed during the evaluation year for each person. Because outcomes could only be measured for older people who received a follow-up interview, those who died or moved away had to be excluded. This left 63 of the matched care scheme cases and 66 of the matched comparison cases for analysis. Because those who had died or moved away did not always constitute matched pairs, the two groups were inevitably no longer quite as well matched as initially.

The outcome predicted was quality of care, expressed as a reduction in need, measured as the improvement in the indicator over the evaluation year. Analysis was undertaken separately for care scheme and comparison cases by means of multiple regression analysis, in which predictors of outcome were drawn from a pool of different initial characteristics and types of resource input. The characteristics included aspects of health and dependency, social support, personality and attitude to help, initial level of well-being and health status, and effect on informal carers. Resources were measured as the number of units of each type of social services department and National Health Service resource consumed during the evaluation year. As helper fees and expenses could not be expressed in units, they were included as monetary units. This pool of possible predictors is summarised in Box 6.1.

### *Care scheme*

The equation predicting reduction in need is shown in Table 6.7. It is clear that initial level of need was the strongest predictor of reduction in need. This may

**Table 6.7**

*Predicting reduction in need for matched care scheme cases who received a follow-up interview*

| Variable | Coefficient | Standard error | p value |
|---|---|---|---|
| *Social support* | | | |
| Support from relatives | 0.16 | 0.05 | 0.002 |
| *Personality and attitude to help* | | | |
| Independent — requires persuasion | 0.97 | 0.47 | 0.046 |
| Passive — dependent attitude | -5.59 | 1.47 | <0.001 |
| *Initial level of well-being* | | | |
| Need | 1.02 | 0.10 | <0.001 |
| *Other client factors* | | | |
| Age of older person | 0.08 | 0.04 | 0.019 |
| Whether female | 2.66 | 0.95 | 0.007 |
| *Resource inputs* | | | |
| Hours of home help | 0.01 | 0.00 | 0.003 |
| Days of day care | 0.03 | 0.01 | 0.002 |
| Days of residential care | 0.03 | 0.01 | 0.006 |
| Hours of care management time | 0.02 | 0.01 | 0.053 |
| Hours of community nursing | 0.01 | 0.00 | 0.030 |
| Constant | -19.51 | 3.22 | <0.001 |

F = 20.3
p value <0.001
$R^2$ = 0.81
Adj. $R^2$ = 0.77
Number of cases = 63

suggest that care managers were achieving the greatest improvements in care with those who needed it the most. Support from relatives was also effective in reducing need, and females were likely to experience a higher reduction in need than males.

A greater reduction was achieved for those who had an independent attitude to help but who would accept some assistance if persuaded, although conversely, those with a passive-dependent attitude to help experienced a lower reduction in need, perhaps being less responsive to care inputs, causing need to increase.

As might be expected, a number of services — home help, day care, nursing and residential care — contributed to reduction in need. Although helper fees did not appear significant, care management time and community nursing were. The association of care manager time with a reduction in need was likely to occur largely through time spent in supporting the care scheme helpers.

Interestingly, the evidence of impact of community services may be associated with their planned coordination through care management.

### Standard provision

It can be seen from Table 6.8 that, as with the care scheme group, initial need was the strongest predictor of its reduction. This suggests a degree of targeting of resources though the effect was not quite as strong as for the care scheme. Older people who were confused or disorientated experienced a greater reduction in need, although this effect did not reach significance ($p = 0.102$). This rather surprising result was probably caused by the greater proportion of older people entering long-term institutional care. The presence of a confidante appeared to lead to greater reductions in need, a finding which is interesting in that previous work has identified the 'protective' qualities of such a relationship more than its propensity to enable gain in well-being (Brown and Harris, 1978).

**Table 6.8**
*Predicting reduction in need for matched comparison cases who received a follow-up interview*

| Variable | Coefficient | Standard error | p value |
|---|---|---|---|
| **Health and dependency** | | | |
| Confusion/disorientation | 0.20 | 0.12 | 0.102 |
| **Social support** | | | |
| Presence of confidant(e) | 1.18 | 0.50 | 0.023 |
| **Initial level of well-being** | | | |
| Need | 0.65 | 0.10 | <0.001 |
| **Other client factors** | | | |
| Bereavement during past year | 1.31 | 0.56 | 0.022 |
| **Resource inputs** | | | |
| Hours of community nursing | 0.03 | 0.01 | 0.012 |
| **Intermediate outcomes** | | | |
| Whether entered long-term institutional care | 4.75 | 0.51 | <0.001 |
| Constant | -4.44 | 1.26 | <0.001 |

$F = 27.87$
$p$ value $<0.001$
$R^2 = 0.74$
Adj. $R^2 = 0.71$
Number of cases = 66

A recent bereavement at first assessment was also associated with reduction in need. This apparently paradoxical observation is likely to be associated with a degree of recovery from the loss by the time of follow-up, which would be more than a year after the event.

In terms of service effects, the major influence of residential care on well-being for comparison group cases, which was noted earlier, was clear. Community services, by contrast with the care scheme, appeared to have little impact on quality of care.

## Conclusion

The care scheme appeared to have been successful in enabling older people to remain in their own homes for longer, and in most cases, avoid entry to long-stay care. The findings suggest that standard domiciliary service provision was ineffective in preventing such admissions for the comparison group, given a substantial number entered long-stay care. Those receiving the care scheme showed improvements in terms both of the quality of the care they received and their quality of life, compared with those in the comparison group. Benefits were also experienced by those older people who entered long-stay care. The worst option from the point of view of the older person was to remain at home and receive standard domiciliary services.

A variety of factors appear to be associated with improved outcomes. However, the range of resource effects evident in the care scheme group would suggest that the impact of services upon well-being is much greater when those services are planned and coordinated in an integrated fashion.

# 7 Outcomes for Carers

The variety of experiences, needs and problems of carers have been recognised for some time, although in recent years there has been a substantial increase in the amount of research and review literature in this area. A study of informal carers based upon General Household Survey data (Green, 1988) estimated that about one adult in seven is involved in looking after an elderly or disabled relative. Overall, 15 per cent of adult females (3.5 million in all) and 12 per cent of adult males (2.5 million in all) defined themselves as carers. This represents about six million carers in all, and the majority (75 per cent) were looking after a person aged 65 and over. It was estimated that one quarter were providing twenty hours and above of care a week, and that 15 per cent were providing 50 hours a week and above. Most carers, three out of four, are women, usually daughters, wives and mothers of their dependants. Most are in middle or late middle age, and growing numbers are themselves elderly (Hicks, 1988). Policy documents have recognised the central role of informal care in the provision of community care. Recent policy documents in the United Kingdom and overseas have recommended that carers' views and needs should be taken into consideration (Griffiths, 1988; Thorslund and Parker, 1994) and the White Paper, *Caring for People*, affirms that practical support for carers should be one of the six key objectives for service delivery (Cm 849, para. 1.1). More recently the importance of carers has been confirmed by the *Carers Act* (1995) and the White Paper, *Modernising Social Services* (Cm 4169, 1998). Underlying this view of the centrality of informal care is the perception that public support for carers represents a long-term investment, a view that is also evident in other countries (Kraan et al., 1991).

Clearly, the substantial amount of informal care provided enables many older people to remain at home. Therefore it was important to examine the effects of the service on the carers of the older people. In this study interviews were undertaken with 71 carers immediately before receipt of the care scheme.

These carers were identified as being substantially involved in providing regular sustained support at the time of the initial assessment. Of those older people with no identified carer, nonetheless, 17 per cent received considerable informal help and a further 76 per cent received a little informal help. Indeed, only two people in receipt of the care scheme had no informal care at all. Interviews were also undertaken with 100 comparison group carers at the point when the older person they supported was identified as a suitable high-need comparison case. Follow-up interviews were undertaken one year later with 40 care scheme carers and 61 comparison group carers.

This chapter examines the extent to which the scheme was successful in alleviating the problems experienced by carers, both to enhance their quality of life and to enable them to continue supporting the older person at home. It begins by describing the carers and their caring role, prior to receipt of the scheme. Second, it examines their experiences of the care scheme service. Finally, the chapter compares the outcomes over time of the carers who received support from the care scheme with those of the comparison group of carers. The analysis of outcomes includes changes in quality of life, and the factors leading to the breakdown of informal care.

## The experience of caring

This section describes the carers. It describes their experiences of caring prior to receipt of the care scheme, including the tasks they performed; the care problems they experienced; other support received, both formal and informal; and the effects of caring, or burdens, on different areas of their life.

Table 7.1 describes the carers. Their mean age was 55 and three-quarters were female, half of whom were daughters or daughters-in-law. A similar proportion, 72 per cent, were married. A low proportion, 14 per cent, actually lived with the person they cared for, reflected in the fact that very few indeed, only three per cent, were spouse carers. In some instances an elderly couple received the care scheme individually in their own right, which may partly account for this low percentage.

Table 7.2 shows the care tasks that the carers performed. A third were involved in helping the person to get up or go to bed, and similarly providing breakfast, on more than one day a week. Just over half prepared other meals on more than one day a week and almost a third prepared tea on almost a daily basis. Almost a quarter were involved in doing light housework tasks on most days of the week. Although only 11 per cent provided personal care on most days, a further 52 per cent provided personal care on some days during the week. For many carers dealing with incontinence as an aspect of personal care was the most unpleasant task they had to carry out. Over half, 61 per cent, of the carers undertook a check-up visit most days. Eighty per cent performed tasks outside the home more than once a week. Just under half spent time for

**Table 7.1**
*Characteristics of the carers*

|  |  | Number | % |
|---|---|---|---|
| Number of carers |  | 71 | - |
| Age of carer | 30 or under | 2 | 3 |
|  | 31–40 | 11 | 16 |
|  | 41–50 | 16 | 22 |
|  | 51–60 | 12 | 17 |
|  | 61–70 | 20 | 28 |
|  | 71–80 | 7 | 10 |
|  | 81 and over | 3 | 4 |
| Mean age |  | 55 | - |
| Gender | male | 18 | 25 |
|  | female | 53 | 75 |
| Marital status | married | 51 | 72 |
|  | single | 8 | 11 |
|  | widowed | 8 | 11 |
|  | separated/divorced | 4 | 6 |
| Whether older person lives with carer |  | 10 | 14 |
| Relationship to older person | husband | 2 | 3 |
|  | son | 5 | 7 |
|  | daughter | 23 | 32 |
|  | daughter-in-law | 4 | 6 |
|  | brother | 3 | 4 |
|  | sister | 2 | 3 |
|  | sister-in-law | 1 | 1 |
|  | other relative — male | 3 | 4 |
|  | — female | 9 | 12 |
|  | unrelated male | 5 | 7 |
|  | unrelated female | 14 | 20 |
| Whether of same generation as older person |  | 17 | 22 |
| Whether children under 16 living at home |  | 13 | 18 |

Not all spouses are carers.
Some spouses receive the scheme in their own right.

companionship on most days. The average number of hours which carers reported was spent on these tasks each week was about 30 hours.

In caring for the older person, the carers experienced a variety of needs and behaviours, both psychological and physical. Many of the problems, shown in Table 7.3, have been found to be poorly tolerated by carers. In particular, problems of incontinence, night disturbance and demanding behaviour have been frequently reported as causing distress to carers (Isaacs, 1971; Sanford, 1975;

**Table 7.2**
*Care tasks*

| Care task | Always/ nearly always % | Sometimes % | Once a week or less % |
|---|---|---|---|
| Help in getting up and going to bed | 16 | 18 | 66 |
| Preparing breakfast | 21 | 13 | 66 |
| Preparing lunch | 17 | 37 | 46 |
| Preparing tea | 32 | 23 | 45 |
| Assisting with light housework | 23 | 42 | 35 |
| Help with personal care or heavy lifting | 11 | 52 | 37 |
| Making regular check up visits | 61 | 28 | 11 |
| Spending time for supervision purposes | 39 | 37 | 24 |
| Providing help away from home: e.g. shopping, outings, gardening | 10 | 70 | 20 |
| Spending time mainly for companionship | 45 | 37 | 18 |

**Table 7.3**
*Older person's behaviour problems*

| Behaviour problem | Constant/ periodic % | Occasional % | None % |
|---|---|---|---|
| *Psychological problems* | | | |
| Dangerous to self or others | 48 | 21 | 31 |
| Uncooperative/personality conflicts | 61 | 25 | 14 |
| Odd speech/unusual ideas/bizarre behaviour | 35 | 27 | 38 |
| Hypochondriasis | 21 | 13 | 66 |
| Demanding excessive companionship | 51 | 11 | 38 |
| Daytime wandering | 4 | 16 | 80 |
| Noisy or wandering at night | 10 | 22 | 68 |
| Deafness/communication difficulties | 23 | 11 | 66 |
| *Physical problems* | | | |
| Requiring nursing or physical care | 77 | 17 | 6 |
| Falling | 73 | 13 | 14 |
| Incontinence of urine | 21 | 37 | 42 |
| Incontinence of faeces | 14 | 35 | 51 |

Greene et al., 1982; Gilleard, 1984; Argyle et al., 1985; Morris, et al., 1988; Levin et al., 1989).

Clearly many carers felt that the older person could not safely be left alone for long periods. Almost half the carers considered the older person a danger to him or herself, or to others. This frequently involved fears about the older person burning kettles, or leaving the gas on. A perception of uncooperative behaviour on the part of the person receiving care was experienced consistently by over 60 per cent of the carers. About half the carers felt the older person was making excessive demands on their time for companionship, and some commented that they seemed to want them to be there all the time. Approximately three-quarters of the carers felt that the older person needed regular nursing care, and a similar proportion were perceived to be at a high risk of falling. Thus, carers experienced a significant amount of both physical care problems and behavioural problems in supporting the older people.

Table 7.4 shows the support and practical help received from carers by family and friends both inside and outside their household. Support received from within the household only includes those carers who lived with other family members, 63 carers, whereas support outside the household includes all 71 carers. Only 25 per cent received regular help in undertaking personal care tasks from within the household, compared with 41 per cent who received such help from family and friends outside the household. Similarly, fewer carers received help with housework and shopping from within the household, 32 per cent compared with 52 per cent (p < 0.05). The area where most support was received by carers, both from within and outside the household,

**Table 7.4**
*Help and support received by carers*

| Support | Intensive/ regular % | Occasional/ never % |
|---|---|---|
| **Help from other family members, relatives or friends within carer's household** | | |
| Personal care | 25 | 75 |
| Housework/shopping | 32 | 68 |
| Moral support | 60 | 40 |
| Number of carers = 63 | | |
| **Help from other family members, relatives or friends outside carer's household** | | |
| Personal care | 41 | 59 |
| Housework/shopping | 52 | 48 |
| Moral support | 66 | 34 |
| Number of carers = 71 | | |
| **Help from statutory agencies** | | |
| Personal care | 65 | 35 |
| Housework/shopping | 78 | 23 |
| Moral support | 66 | 34 |
| Number of carers = 71 | | |

was in terms of moral support, 60 and 66 per cent respectively. Although practical help has been shown to be greatly valued by carers (Challis et al., 1995), this was not received to any great extent by carers from within their household. Assistance for carers in ensuring that personal care tasks and household tasks were undertaken came mainly from statutory agencies, predominately the home help and nursing services.

It is clear that carers experience a variety of costs, both financial through loss of employment (Wright, 1983), and through burdens or the effects on various areas of their life and on their physical and mental health. These burdens have been attributed to caring (Grad and Sainsbury, 1965, 1968; Gilleard et al., 1984; Levin et al., 1989; Parker, 1990; Challis et al., 1995). Table 7.5 examines the burdens experienced by the carers in this study. It is clear that they experienced difficulties and restrictions in their day-to-day routines, social relationships and physical and psychological well-being. The majority, 79 per cent, of carers experienced moderate or severe problems with their household routine. This mainly involved disruptions or changes in their usual shopping and mealtime routines. Three carers had given up full-time jobs to care. In terms of effects on their social life, almost three-quarters of the carers experienced moderate or severe restrictions. Only fourteen of the carers had children living at home, and only one experienced severe problems. Almost one third of the carers felt that their physical health had been severely affected due to caring and 27 per cent felt that their mental health had been severely affected. This is reflected in the malaise score. A cut-off point between four and five on the malaise scale, out of a possible score of 24 was used to identify carers experiencing significant levels of stress (Rutter et al., 1970). This indicated that 68 per cent of the carers were experiencing a high level of stress, which was also evident in the mean score of 8.1.

**Table 7.5**
*Overall ratings of the different types of burdens experienced by carers*

| Burden | None/slight % | Moderate % | Severe % |
|--------|------|------|------|
| Household routine | 21 | 44 | 35 |
| Employment | 72 | 25 | 3 |
| Social life | 28 | 45 | 27 |
| Children | 85 | 14 | 1 |
| Physical health | 30 | 39 | 31 |
| Mental health | 16 | 58 | 27 |

### The experience of the care scheme over time

The carers' experience of the care scheme provides a picture of how services could affect their capacity to cope. This is based upon information from the follow-up interviews at one year. Carers were asked about the effect of the scheme on them as well as on the older person they cared for. Forty carers who had received the support of the scheme were interviewed. In this group of carers, 32 of the older people were still being cared for at home, and eight had been admitted to long-term institutional care during the year.

Three-quarters of the carers said they were doing less than a year ago, whilst only 15 per cent said they were doing more. For those carers who were caring for someone at home this was 68 per cent and 19 per cent respectively. Almost all the carers felt that the scheme had been of help to them during the year. One carer supporting her grandmother, commented, 'I'm so grateful. If it hadn't been for the scheme, she'd have been in a home, against her will, and I'd have had a nervous breakdown.' Others were full of praise for the extensive help received from the scheme, including extra visits and helpers bringing food from their own homes. Carers commented how it enabled them to continue with their lives. A daughter caring for her mother commented, 'It's given me peace of mind'. She was able to continue with her job without worrying about her mother. Another carer, a woman supporting a neighbour, commented that the scheme had rendered a harassing and oppressive situation a tolerable one. She could now go to work knowing that her neighbour would not 'summon' her.

Other positive comments were made about the scheme in enabling care to continue at home by preventing crises from occurring. A woman caring for her father-in-law commented, 'Without the scheme he would have no effective care most of the time. There would have been continued crises with neighbours becoming involved unwillingly and the warden getting agitated.' Another, a married woman caring for her mother, said, 'I cannot describe how much it helped. I don't think I could have gone on the way I was going on'. Although her mother was now in hospital, the scheme had relieved her of weekend visits and of constant phone calls. She felt the scheme enabled her to retain her own health, having previously been in a state of physical and mental collapse due to constant demands.

In fact only one carer said the scheme had not been a help. This was due to her mother having spent almost the entire year in some form of institutional care, due to increasing physical and mental frailty. Two carers had mixed views: one was caring for a friend and had little or no contact with the scheme, limited knowledge about what the scheme did and therefore did not see it as providing any support to her personally; the second, a man caring for a friend, mainly provided friendship, and similarly had little knowledge about what the scheme provided. He said that he would have done the same regardless of the scheme's input.

The carers were asked about the ways in which the care scheme had been successful in providing help to them personally. Eighty-five per cent of the carers stated that it had relieved them of certain tasks or commitments, and some commented how it had enabled them to go out and thus improve their quality of life; 70 per cent said the scheme performed tasks that had previously been neglected; 87 per cent felt it had provided them with relief from the worry or responsibility of caring; 80 per cent said that it provided them with moral support; and 87 per cent were relieved that it provided an improved quality of life for the older person. Several carers commented that the older person let helpers from the scheme do things that he or she would not let the carer do. One carer, supporting his sister described how helpers had succeeded in getting her to accept help she wouldn't take from her family. In general, she did not get on well with anyone due to her mental deterioration, which had made her abusive to everyone, 'They're virtually the only outsiders who come and make a fuss of her'. Furthermore, the input of practical help, shared responsibility, interest and friendship to the family had made the difference between coping and not coping. Significantly, 82 per cent of the carers felt that the service had reduced the risk of entry to residential care.

There were however, some drawbacks associated with the scheme for a minority of older people and their carers. These were mainly concerns which arose when the service was introduced, and were principally centred around strangers coming into the house. One carer described how the friend she cared for made herself ill with worry about strangers coming in and therefore found it hard to accept at first. However, once she got used to the helper these initial anxieties receded and she was content. Several commented that the introduction of the scheme was seen by the older person as an intrusion into their privacy. These reservations were overcome in the main. Such concerns underline the importance of introducing the service at a pace which was acceptable to both the older person and their carer. This is illustrated by one daughter caring for her mother, who commented how her mother had not taken to some helpers at first, but that the helpers overcame this by being flexible and willing to provide care in ways that reflected precisely what her mother wanted. The ability to provide services in a flexible way was clearly important (Challis et al., 1995).

Seventy-nine per cent of the carers reported getting on well with the helpers, 13 per cent gave a mixed response and got on with some better than others, and 8 per cent reported little contact. Most saw helpers at least weekly. One woman caring for her mother who had eventually been admitted to a home, commented, 'The helpers were marvellous. They would do anything.' Sixty-eight per cent reported getting on well with the care manager involved, 18 per cent had little contact and 13 per cent had mixed feelings or did not get on too well with the care manager. Many carers commented that the service had fulfilled and exceeded any expectations they had had, especially in terms of the amount of time given and patience shown to the older person.

Carers were asked whether the scheme had affected their relationship with the older person. Seventy per cent said that their relationship had not been affected. One carer, a nephew caring for his aunt, commented, 'Nothing has altered. She has always been a treasure. She never asks for anything from life.' Another, a daughter caring for her mother, said, 'Nothing would change that, I've always idolised my mother'. One daughter reported that she and her mother had always had a bad relationship and that despite the benefits of the scheme, no amount of help and support would stop her hating her mother, 'If the scheme had not rescued me from mother's constant demands, I would have demanded that she be placed in care'. Thus, the scheme had not affected longstanding features of their relationship, but it had enabled the carer to escape from some of the excessive demands to live her own life. Where the relationship had changed, carers commented that it had improved due to the support of the scheme, relieving the carer, and thus reducing the tension in the relationship. Another daughter commented on the reduction of interpersonal tension. She said 'I can now be fond of my mother. Previously I could cheerfully have killed her when she was being so difficult at home.'

When carers were asked whether or not they felt the older person would be better off in long-term care, of the 32 still at home, 65 per cent said no, 25 per cent said yes and 10 per cent were unsure. Some carers were adamant that the person they cared for would not be happy in long-term care, 'She wouldn't be happy anywhere else'. Another commented, 'She wouldn't cope in a home. She wouldn't live for five minutes in such a place. She might be better off in terms of physical care, but mentally she couldn't stand it.' Other carers commented that they thought the older person would be better off in care, but recognised and respected their wishes to remain in their own home. One carer commented that due to her mother's mental deterioration and need for constant attention she would be better off and safer in long-term care, but recognised that her mother did not wish to enter care and found the scheme a good second best, which had made both her and her mother's situation manageable. This may reflect the greater ability of carers to accept residential care, when mental deterioration is evident (Levin et al., 1989). There was also the recognition for some carers that the only alternative would be hospital care, because the person was now too frail to be admitted into residential care. One son caring for his mother said that without the scheme she would have had to go into care. He still thought that would be the best place for her, both for her own safety and his and his wife's freedom to enjoy their retirement. This carer commented how he repeatedly tried to talk her into accepting care, but the responses were, 'You want rid of me', and, 'I'll soon be gone'. The carer commented, 'She's been saying that for 20 years and is still alive and still a burden'. He felt he had repaid the care she had given him many times over.

## Coping mechanisms

Some studies have recognised the importance of, and attempted to tease out, strategies or coping mechanisms uses by carers (Pearlin and Schooler, 1978; Billings and Moos, 1981; Milne et al., 1993). Carers were asked specific questions about their patterns of coping with the pressures occasioned by supporting the older person. The different methods used by the carers receiving different services were compared. Carers of people in receipt of the care scheme were more frequently able to take holidays away from home and tended to spend more evenings out. Possibly as a consequence, fewer found it necessary to adopt strategies such as overlooking some aspects of the older person's behaviour. Moreover, these carers found it less necessary to talk things over when there were conflicting opinions. These findings suggest that in addition to older people obtaining more relief through the scheme, the level of support provided meant behaviour problems were rendered more manageable for the carers.

## The outcomes of caring

The benefits of the scheme to the carer were determined in a similar way to those for the older people. Outcomes could be calculated when the carer had had both an initial and a follow-up interview. This was normally the case for older people who had remained at home or entered institutional care. However, when the older person had died, the follow-up interview was not carried out for ethical reasons. Follow-up interviews were carried out with 40 care scheme carers and 61 comparison group carers. An outcome was treated as the difference between an indicator at the initial interview and its value at follow-up. Analysis of variance was then used to compare changes in quality of life between care scheme and comparison groups.

As in the case of the outcomes for older people discussed in the previous chapter, the effect of whether or not the older person was admitted to institutional care was examined as well as that of experimental/comparison group. It is clear that an admission to institutional care would have a major impact on the carer's situation. As with the outcome measurement for older people, matched groups were not used. Any differences between the groups at initial interview were controlled for using covariance analysis.

## Care tasks performed

There were only two significant differences between the two groups of carers in the changes in the frequencies with which care tasks were performed, which involved helping get the older person up and put them to bed ($p < 0.05$), and helping with personal care or heavy lifting ($p < 0.01$). For both of these tasks, whereas the frequency increased over time for the comparison group, it decreased for the care scheme group. These were tasks that were frequently undertaken by the helpers to relieve carers. This was accompanied by a corresponding and significant ($p < 0.05$) increase in the amount of assistance provided by social services in the area of personal care for those cases receiving the new service. Hence, it is clear that, at least at the margin, the scheme supported carers by substituting some of their input with additional services. As would be expected, admission to institutional care led to a significant reduction in all forms of informal carer support except provision of companionship, as the carer normally continued to visit the older person socially although no longer providing physical care.

### Older person's behaviour

The changes reported by carers in patterns of behaviour are shown in Table 7.6. For many aspects of behaviour, it appeared that admission to institutional care reduced the perceived pressure of the problems. This was the case in the areas of dangerous behaviour, uncooperative behaviour, demanding excessive companionship and nocturnal wandering or noise. Risks arising from falling were also reduced from the carers' point of view by the older person's entry to institutional care. However, the scheme was still able to provide carers with a significant reduction in problems caused by uncooperative behaviour and the need for nursing or physical care. Interestingly, both for dangerous and uncooperative behaviours there was also an interaction effect, where clearly the least beneficial option appeared to be to remain at home receiving the usual range of services.

### The burdens of caring

This section considers the ways in which caring for the older person affected different aspects of the carer's life. These costs or burdens of caring are shown in Table 7.7. Although carers of older people receiving the care scheme experienced a greater reduction in problems connected with different aspects of household routine, these effects were statistically insignificant. However admissions to institutional care did lead to a significant reduction in these problems. The number of carers with young children was very small and as a consequence, neither receipt of the scheme nor admission to institutional care appeared to have had any significant effect upon any difficulties associated with their care.

Although there was no significant effect of the scheme on the employment of the carer, it was effective in reducing significantly the adverse effects upon the employment of the carer's spouse, usually the husband. This reflected the pattern of relationships of many of the carers. Admission to institutional care

**Table 7.6**
*Carer outcomes: older person's behaviour problems*

| | | Mean | | Tests | |
|---|---|---|---|---|---|
| | | E | C | EvC | HvI |
| **Psychological problems** | | | | | |
| Dangerous to self or others | Home: | -0.3 | 0.1 | ns* | <0.001 |
| | Inst: | -0.9 | -1.3 | | |
| Uncooperative/personality conflicts | Home: | -0.2 | 0.2 | <0.01* | <0.01 |
| | Inst: | -1.3 | -0.1 | | |
| Demanding excessive companionship | Home: | -0.1 | 0.1 | ns | <0.01 |
| | Inst: | -0.5 | -0.7 | | |
| Daytime wandering | Home: | -0.2 | -0.1 | ns | ns |
| | Inst: | -0.1 | -0.1 | | |
| Noisy or wandering at night | Home: | -0.3 | 0.1 | ns | <0.01 |
| | Inst: | -0.4 | -0.6 | | |
| **Physical problems** | | | | | |
| Requiring nursing or physical care | Home: | -0.2 | 0.3 | <0.05 | ns |
| | Inst: | -0.1 | 0.0 | | |
| Falling | Home: | -0.1 | -0.1 | ns | <0.01 |
| | Inst: | -0.6 | -0.9 | | |
| Incontinence of urine | Home: | -0.1 | 0.1 | ns | ns |
| | Inst: | -0.3 | -0.1 | | |
| Incontinence of faeces | Home: | 0.1 | 0.1 | ns | ns |
| | Inst: | 0.0 | -0.1 | | |

E = experimental group (number of cases = 40); C = comparison group (number of cases = 61)
H = home (at one year); I = institution (at one year).
ns = not significant.
\* = significant interaction effect.

resulted, naturally, in a reduction in the overall effect on employment of both the carer and spouse (p = 0.07).

The care scheme was successful in reducing disruption to a variety of aspects of social life, mainly through providing relief. Thus, a significantly greater number felt more able to have visitors (p < 0.01) and to have holidays (p < 0.01), as well as engaging in more social activities. Admission to institutional care led to a dramatic improvement in the opportunity to participate in all aspects of social life, as might be expected. Overall, carers of people receiving the care scheme experienced less interference with social life (p = 0.06), an effect that was almost significant. Admission to institutional care led to improvements in many areas of the carer's social life: visiting friends (p < 0.01); going out (p < 0.05); more social activities (p < 0.05); having visitors (p < 0.05);

**Table 7.7**
*Carer outcomes: burdens of caring*

| | | Mean | | Tests | |
|---|---|---|---|---|---|
| | | E | C | EvC | HvI |
| Household routine | Home: | -0.5 | -0.2 | ns | <0.001 |
| | Inst: | -1.1 | -1.0 | | |
| Employment | Home: | -0.2 | -0.2 | ns | ns |
| | Inst: | -0.6 | -0.3 | | |
| Social life | Home: | -0.5 | -0.1 | ns | ns |
| | Inst: | -0.8 | -0.8 | | |
| Physical health | Home: | -0.5 | -0.1 | <0.05 | ns |
| | Inst: | -0.8 | -0.5 | | |
| Mental health | Home: | -0.6 | 0.0 | <0.001 | ns |
| | Inst: | -0.5 | -0.5 | | |
| Expressed burden | Home: | -0.6 | -0.1 | <0.05 | <0.01 |
| | Inst: | -0.8 | -0.8 | | |

E = experimental group (number of cases = 40); C = comparison group (number of cases = 61)
H = home (at one year); I = institution (at one year).
ns = not significant.

more time spent with spouse (p < 0.05); and more holidays (p < 0.001). However, the overall effect was not significant.

As well as the effects on the carer's lifestyle, it is important to consider how the physical and emotional health of the carer was effected by the new service. The scheme was effective in significantly reducing the carer's physical health difficulties. An admission to institutional care also appeared to reduce these health problems, although the finding was not significant. Receipt of the care scheme service also successfully reduced some aspects of the carer's mental health difficulties. Table 7.7 shows that overall mental health pressures were reduced for the carers receiving the scheme. This is particularly important given the general recognition that the greatest cost to carers is in terms of the effects on their psychological health (Grad and Sainsbury, 1965; Isaacs et al., 1972; Gilleard, 1984; Gilleard et al., 1984; Levin et al., 1989). Specific elements of this, feelings of anxiety and worry were significantly reduced. For those remaining at home, carers of older people receiving the care scheme became much less anxious, while in the comparison group there was little change. Where older people had entered institutional care, carers experienced a reduction in anxiety, presumably as a result of relief from the commitment of caring. Sleeping problems were noted less frequently and adverse effects on other family members were also significantly smaller for those receiving the care scheme. The scheme also appeared to be successful in enabling the carer to relax more (p = 0.06).

Admission to institutional care also appeared to lead to improvement in the carer's mental health overall although this was not quite statistically significant. This reflects the findings of others (Whittick, 1985; Gibbins, 1986; Levin et al., 1989). Most interestingly, the only group not to experience an improvement in mental health consisted of carers of older people in the comparison group who remained in the community.

Carers of older people receiving the care scheme experienced a significantly greater reduction in the sense of burden associated with providing support. The reduction in burden where the person entered institutional care was also significant (Brown et al., 1990). Again it is noteworthy that those carers receiving standard services at home benefited least.

### Summary outcome indicators

The findings from a series of summary outcome indicators are shown in Table 7.8. These cover carer inputs, behaviour problems, lifestyle including social and domestic routines, strain, tension and psychological distress or malaise. There was clearly a significant reduction in the amount of care given when the older person had been admitted to care in both groups, indicating the effect of institutional provision upon the demands made on carers. However, whereas for those at home receiving the scheme there was a small reduction in

**Table 7.8**
*Carer outcomes: summary indicators*

|  |  | Mean | | Tests | |
|---|---|---|---|---|---|
|  |  | E | C | EvC | HvI |
| Change in amount of care given | Home: | -1.6 | 1.5 | ns | <0.001 |
|  | Inst: | -21.3 | -26.0 |  |  |
| Behaviour problems | Home: | -1.6 | 1.0 | <0.05 | <0.001 |
|  | Inst: | -4.8 | -3.7 |  |  |
| Lifestyle problems | Home: | -1.8 | -0.7 | 0.05 | <0.001 |
|  | Inst: | -3.4 | -2.8 |  |  |
| Level of strain | Home: | -1.0 | -0.1 | <0.001 | <0.001 |
|  | Inst: | -1.8 | -1.2 |  |  |
| Level of tension in home | Home: | -0.4 | 0.0 | ns | ns |
|  | Inst: | -0.3 | -0.5 |  |  |
| Malaise | Home: | -1.3 | -0.5 | ns | 0.07 |
|  | Inst: | -2.6 | -1.9 |  |  |

E = experimental group (number of cases = 40); C = comparison group (number of cases = 61)
H = home (at one year); I = institution (at one year).
ns = not significant.

demands upon carers, for those carers in the comparison group there was a small increase in the demands made on them. An aggregated indicator of behaviour problems showed that carers of people receiving the care scheme as well as those admitted to institutional care experienced significantly fewer problems. Those comparison group carers receiving standard services at home fared worst.

When the effects on different aspects of the carer's lifestyle and their physical health were combined into an overall rating, this indicated a statistically significant improvement in the case of both the care scheme and institutional care. This was also the case with an aggregate rating of strain.

The overall level of stress experienced by the carers was measured by means of the Malaise Scale (Rutter et al., 1970). Although carers of older people receiving the care scheme experienced a greater reduction in malaise, this effect was not statistically significant. However, admission to institutional care did appear to reduce the level of malaise ($p = 0.07$). Rutter et al. (1970), in their work with mothers of handicapped and mentally ill children, identified a score of over 4 as indicating significant stress. In view of the high stress levels evident in the present group, a score of 7 or over was treated as severe stress. Using this indicator, it is noteworthy that of those individuals with a critical level of stress at the first interview, whereas only 12 per cent of the comparison group carers improved to a point below this threshold, 25 per cent of those carers receiving the scheme did so. There was an almost significant reduction in stress for those carers when the older person they cared for entered institutional care ($p = 0.07$).

It is interesting to note which items of this scale appeared to be contributing to the differences. Some aspects of physical symptoms of anxiety appeared to reduce for those receiving the scheme. Entry of the older person to institutional care was associated with factors such as improvement in the carer's appetite. Further corroboratory evidence of the reduction in stress of admission to institutional care can be found (McKay et al., 1983; Levin et al., 1989, 1994).

## Welfare gain in quality of life of carers

In the previous chapter the concept of 'welfare gain' was formulated to allow for the temporal effect on welfare. This was based upon the concept of 'Health Gain' (Cm 1523, 1992). In this an attempt was made to take account of the gain experienced from different types of provision, care management or standard provision, by attempting to allow for the levels of well-being at intermediate stages of the evaluation year.

A full picture could of course only be obtained from knowledge of the level of well-being at all times during the period, which was not feasible. However, a simple approach was developed which rested on the evidence of difference between different types of setting in their impact upon outcomes. Earlier in the chapter the differences between the level of well-being for those at home and in institutional care for both experimental and comparison groups was noted. Some allowance could be made for these fluctuations by assuming that the mean value of improvement in well-being for those who remained at home was representative of all periods spent at home for all, while the corresponding value for those who moved into institutional care was representative of all periods spent in institutional care, with experimental and comparison groups being considered separately. Welfare gain over the year could then be estimated by weighting the improvement in outcome while at home by the average period spent at home and adding the improvement in outcome while in institutional care weighted by the average period spent in institutional care.

In the analysis of outcomes for carers the effect of the concept of welfare gain was, as previously, to increase the extent of the effect between those receiving the scheme and the comparison group. Again, this was attributable to the poorest outcome effect being that of remaining at home and receiving existing services for the comparison group. The benefits were particularly evident with regard to effects on household routine and social life for carers. This care scheme effect was to some extent offset for carers, in comparison to the older people, by the higher probability of the person being admitted to institutional care in the comparison group and the gains which carers experienced as a consequence.

Thus, if it is possible to view well-being more as a quantity of welfare produced through time than the cross-sectional comparisons discussed earlier, the effect could well be to increase the positive effects of the care management approach. Of course, it would be desirable to examine this approach with more appropriate data collected at more frequent intervals so as to make it less reliant on the assumptions outlined above. Measures of outcome of social care interventions which take account of the time period through which benefits are enjoyed, as well as the apparent benefits of the intervention, may prove to be more sensitive and more appropriate as a basis for decisions about the allocation of resources, in the same way as indicators of disability and ill health have been combined to produce indicators of disability adjusted life years (Murray et al., 1993).

In examining outcomes for carers it has frequently been the case that it is the carers of older people in the comparison group who are not admitted to institutional care who benefit least. This is the same group for which the older person's outcomes were least favourable. Thus, it would seem that if community-based care is to have an impact upon carers' needs, it must be both more intensive and flexible than existing services have hitherto proved to be. Furthermore, in some situations of extreme stress, even highly responsive community-based care may be unable to provide the degree of relief to carers that is offered by residential or nursing home care. It is at this point that the delicate balance of potentially conflicting needs of the older person and the carer needs to be addressed explicitly.

It is clear from the results of outcomes for carers that on the whole the scheme was effective in reducing stress and improving quality of life. In the next section the reasons why some carers withdrew from their caring role are investigated.

## Factors precipitating breakdown of carer support

It has been noted that one essential source of help in assisting many frail older people to stay at home is the informal care network, and that a function of enhanced community care is to support carers. When faced by too many problems, a breakdown in this means of support may occur. It is clearly useful to know which are the factors which are most likely to lead to withdrawal of the carer. These are examined in this section.

### Definition of breakdown

Although it is frequently not possible to pin-point any one factor as causing breakdown of informal support at home, problems experienced by the carer are clearly important (Booth, undated; Levin et al., 1989, 1994). Also, as an older person finds it increasingly difficult to manage at home through deteriorating health and ability to cope, they may take the initiative in seeking institutional care. Alternatively they may have, through ill health or a crisis such as a fall, to be admitted to acute hospital care.

For these analyses, it was assumed that where the primary factor causing the older person to leave home was acute illness, they were not regarded as having left through a breakdown in the carer's support, since following treatment they would be expected to be discharged home. Older people who left home to enter long-term residential or hospital care were regarded as having left due to a breakdown in the care network, where such a network existed, whereas those who remained at home were regarded as having carers who had continued in their supportive role.

All cases in both groups with a carer who had been interviewed were used as a basis for this analysis. The rate of breakdown was significantly different for the two groups, with far fewer of the care scheme cases entering care, eight (11 per cent), compared with 37 (37 per cent) of the comparison group cases ($p < 0.001$).

Those factors included which might influence breakdown were confined to the situation at the time of the initial assessment, and three types were examined: those concerning the older person; those concerning the carer; and those concerning the interrelationship between the two. These variables are listed in Box 7.1.

Logistic regression analysis was used to predict the probability of the breakdown of care. This is a multivariate technique designed to predict the

**Box 7.1**
*Variables used in predicting carer breakdown*

**Carer factors**
Age of carer
Gender of carer
Whether caring for more than 1 year
Whether carer is married to older person
Whether carer is related to older person but not spouse
Number of carer's children under 16 if living with older person
Number of carer's children under 16 if not living with older person
Carer married, living with older person and no children
Carer married, not living with older person and with no children
Whether carer unmarried and living with older person
Degree of carer stress (malaise score)
Whether carer gives regular personal care
Effects on carer's lifestyle:
    extent of interference with household routine
    extent of interference with employment
    extent of interference with social life
    extent of interference with children
    sometimes/frequently suffers backstrain through lifting

**Older person factors**
Gender of older person
Dependence score at times of rising and retiring
Dependence score with other personal care tasks
Whether needs help with bathing
Whether needs help with meal preparation
Whether needs help in preparing a hot drink or a snack
Frequent/total incontinence of urine
Frequent/total incontinence of faeces
Whether at severe risk of falling
Whether lonely often/most of the time
Wakefield depression score
Whether moderately/severely confused

**Older person/carer interactions and relationship factors**
Presence of polarisation among informal carers
Presence of positive communication expressed toward older person
Hostility expressed toward older person
High level of expressed emotion in carer
Presence of behaviour problems:
    dangerous to self or others
    wilfully uncooperative/personality conflicts
    uses odd speech, expresses unusual ideas, 'bizarre' behaviour
    hypochondriasis
    requiring nursing or physical care
    demanding excessive companionship
    daytime wandering
    noisy or wandering at night
    deafness/communication difficulties

probability of a binary outcome, in this case breakdown or non-breakdown of care. Each group is examined separately below.

*Factors predicting breakdown amongst carers of older people in the comparison group*

A large number of indicators contributed towards carer breakdown amongst the comparison group. These are shown in Table 7.9. A fairly high proportion of the variance could now be explained, with 81 per cent correct predictions of breakdown.

Turning first to carer factors, it can be seen female carers were more likely to give up the caring role than male carers and that certain types of relative or family care arrangements were more likely to lead to breakdown. Thus relatives of the older person and particularly spouses were more likely to withdraw. The number of children under 16 also influenced the likelihood of the carer giving up (Gilhooly, 1986). Also married carers living away from the older person were more likely to give up, whether or not they had children under 16 at home. This finding is consistent with that of Argyle et al. (1985) for carers of psychogeriatric patients who could no longer cope.

Interference with employment was significantly associated with a reduced likelihood of breakdown. This implies that carers who had given up their job or reduced their hours of working in order to devote themselves to caring for the older person were less likely to give up. Interestingly, those whose physical health was affected were more likely to continue caring. As might be expected, effects on mental health were likely to lead to the breakdown of care (Zarit et al., 1986; Gilleard 1987; Jerrom et al., 1993). However, high stress scores, as measured by the malaise scale (Rutter et al., 1990), were to some extent associated with a reduced likelihood of carer breakdown, although this was not statistically significant (p = 0.096). Thus carers with the capacity to continue caring appeared to be able to tolerate a degree of physical ill-health and general stress, though specific evidence of mental health problems was unsurprisingly more likely to lead to breakdown of support.

In considering factors associated with the older person, it might appear surprising that, although the care of those needing help with getting up and going to bed was more likely to break down, those needing help with other personal care tasks such as toileting, feeding and transfer and those needing help with bathing were less likely to experience breakdown of informal support. This result occurred despite the fact that when the carer was involved in helping with personal care, this increased the likelihood of breakdown. These are of course more likely to be the kind of activities where services can substitute or complement the carer's role, unlike early morning and late evening support. Hence need for these forms of care might indicate areas where services could be effective. Conversely, where the carers themselves were providing the personal care, the probability of breakdown appeared greater. Care was also

**Table 7.9**
*Older person and carer factors predicting the breakdown of care for the comparison group*

| Variable | Coefficient | Std error | Wald statistic[a] | p value |
|---|---|---|---|---|
| **Carer factors** | | | | |
| Gender of carer (whether female) | | | | |
| Carer married to older person | 1.67 | 0.94 | 3.14 | 0.076 |
| Carer related to older person, not spouse | 5.90 | 2.29 | 6.65 | 0.010 |
| No. of children < 16, not living with older | 2.36 | 1.12 | 4.42 | 0.036 |
| person | 1.78 | 0.74 | 5.74 | 0.017 |
| Married, no children, living with older person | | | | |
| Married, no children, not living with older | -3.90 | 2.32 | 2.82 | 0.093 |
| person | 1.94 | 0.90 | 4.69 | 0.030 |
| Effect upon employment | | | | |
| Effect upon physical health | -1.84 | 0.74 | 6.29 | 0.012 |
| Effect upon mental health | -1.96 | 0.76 | 6.75 | 0.009 |
| Carer stress | 1.93 | 0.94 | 4.20 | 0.041 |
| | -0.17 | 0.10 | 2.77 | 0.096 |
| **Older person factors** | | | | |
| Needing help with getting up and going to bed | | | | |
| Needing help with toileting, feeding, transfer | 0.63 | 0.38 | 2.81 | 0.094 |
| Needing help with bathing | -2.20 | 0.70 | 9.87 | 0.002 |
| At severe risk of falling | -2.64 | 1.10 | 5.76 | 0.016 |
| | 1.67 | 0.97 | 2.99 | 0.084 |
| **Older person/carer interactions and relationship factors** | | | | |
| Carer gives regular personal care | | | | |
| Dangerous to self or others | 3.40 | 0.96 | 12.62 | <0.001 |
| Deafness or communication difficulties | 1.65 | 0.85 | 3.77 | 0.052 |
| Polarisation of care | -1.58 | 0.76 | 4.37 | 0.037 |
| Carer hostility towards older person | 1.35 | 0.89 | 2.33 | 0.127 |
| | 3.65 | 1.41 | 6.73 | 0.010 |
| Constant | | | | |
| | -5.56 | 2.10 | 7.01 | 0.008 |

Correct predictions = 81%
Goodness of fit chi-squared = 73.89
p value = 0.671
df = 80

a The Wald statistic is the coefficient divided by the standard error, squared. Under the hypothesis of a zero coefficient, it has a chi-squared distribution with one degree of freedom.

somewhat more likely to break down for those older people who were at severe risk of falling, although this result was not statistically significant (p = 0.084). Argyle et al. (1985) reported a similar finding.

Problems in the older person/carer relationship were again important predictors of breakdown. As noted, carers providing regular personal care were, in the absence of the care scheme support, more likely to withdraw. Dangerous behaviour on the part of the older person was also likely to cause breakdown. However, deafness or communication difficulties were associated with a reduced risk of breakdown. Carers who were not being helped out by others in the informal network were predictably more likely to withdraw (Ratna and Davis, 1984), though this result was not a significant factor. However, when hostility was expressed towards the older person, this was strongly and significantly associated with breakdown, indicating the difficulties of care-giving where there is a negative relationship between the parties involved.

*Factors predicting breakdown amongst carers of older people receiving the care scheme*

The results of a similar analysis to predict breakdown for those receiving the care scheme are shown in Table 7.10. This equation proved to predict breakdown very effectively, with 96 per cent correct predictions using only seven variables. It must be remembered however, that this analysis included only a small number of carers. Carers whose mental health was suffering were, like those in the comparison group, more likely to withdraw, a similar finding to

**Table 7.10**
*Older person and carer factors predicting the breakdown of care for those receiving the care scheme service*

| Variable | Coefficient | Std error | Wald statistic[a] | p value |
|---|---|---|---|---|
| **Carer factors** | | | | |
| Extent of interference with mental health | 10.83 | 5.45 | 3.94 | 0.047 |
| **Older person factors** | | | | |
| Gender of older person (whether female) | -12.67 | 6.22 | 4.16 | 0.042 |
| Depressed state | 0.58 | 0.28 | 4.38 | 0.036 |
| **Older person/carer interactions and relationship factors** | | | | |
| Demanding excessive companionship | -7.76 | 4.18 | 3.45 | 0.063 |
| Daytime wandering | 9.64 | 4.71 | 4.19 | 0.041 |
| Deafness/communication difficulties | 6.23 | 3.77 | 2.75 | 0.098 |
| High level of carer emotion | 6.92 | 3.14 | 4.87 | 0.027 |
| Constant | -11.07 | 7.42 | 2.23 | 0.136 |

Correct predictions = 96%
Goodness of fit chi-squared = 16.98
p value = 1
df = 63

a The Wald statistic is the coefficient divided by the standard error, squared. Under the hypothesis of a zero coefficient, it has a chi-squared distribution with one degree of freedom.

that of Argyle et al. (1985) for carers suffering anxiety or depression. However the higher stress score and health problems associated with comparison group carers who continued caring were not found for these carers. This may illustrate one way in which the scheme may have impacted upon the quality of life of carers, by at least reducing the stress for these individuals.

In terms of characteristics of the older people, males were significantly more likely to have a carer withdraw than females. Also depression in the older person was associated with breakdown in informal care.

In terms of the older person/carer relationship, daytime wandering and a high level of emotion in the carer significantly contributed towards breakdown (Vaughn and Leff, 1976). Deafness or communication difficulties were associated with breakdown, perhaps because support from helpers would be more difficult to establish. Although older people who demand excessive companionship are a well-known cause of carer stress, they were surprisingly associated with maintenance of carer support.

So once again, older person/carer relationship problems were important factors leading to breakdown of care. Problems of mental health in the carer and depression in the older person were both significant factors contributing towards the withdrawal of informal support. Also carers of males were more likely to give up providing support.

### Caring and the breakdown of care

In these analyses it was only possible to begin to tease out the complexity of factors associated with breakdown of care. In analyses of both those receiving the care scheme and those receiving the usual range of services, it was apparent that not only were the particular individual characteristics of the older person and the carer important, but also the way in which they interact, which may reflect the quality of the relationship. Clearly what is important for services to support carers is to begin to identify ways in which the more stressful or negative features of such a relationship may be alleviated, and also to identify where such elements may be so longstanding that no such relief is feasible or perhaps desirable. One step towards this could be the development of typologies of such relationships. For example, Bergmann (1979) developed an analysis of breakdown of caring relationships through a focus on disequilibriating factors. This was based upon analysis of the relative power, autonomy and rewardingness which could be deployed by the older person in the context of family relationships.

### Conclusion

Carers tended to be very satisfied with the support they received from the scheme, and at follow-up were undertaking fewer tasks in care than when first seen. This was quite different from the experience of those carers receiving the usual range of domiciliary care services, for whom the amount of care-giving tended to increase. The analyses of outcomes for carers present a consistent pattern, not dissimilar in many ways from those for the older people themselves. Carers appeared to benefit both from receiving the scheme, or when the older person entered long-stay care. However, it appeared that the least helpful option for carers was to continue receiving the limited support offered from standard domiciliary services. If services are to maintain frail older people at home and provide adequate support to carers they need to be focused, coordinated, intensive and flexible.

# 8   Costs and Outcomes of Care

This chapter examines the costs of care for the care scheme and comparison groups in the study. Cost data was collected on the flow of resources over a 12 month period from the time at which an older person first received care from the scheme until the 12 month follow-up date, and for a similar period for individuals in the comparison group. For the sake of convenience in standardising all the figures in this study, the price base that has been used in calculating cost figures is 1981-82, the first full year in which the original project was in operation. The first part of the chapter provides a brief overview of the underlying principles upon which the collection of cost data was based. The second part describes briefly the individual unit costs for different services. The third section provides descriptive material and comparative material on the costs to different parties for both the care scheme and comparison groups. In the final section an examination is made of factors which influence variations in costs to major interest groups, defined here as society as a whole and the main agencies. These analyses are important not only for their predictive value in identifying the determinants of costs but also for the descriptive feel which they provide for the ways in which costs were higher or lower according to certain need generating characteristics.

## Costing principles

The approach which was used in providing unit costs for care services was based upon one used in similar evaluative studies in Kent and Darlington (Challis and Davies, 1986; Challis et al., 1993, 1995). Accordingly, less detail of specific calculations is given here. There were three broad principles underlying this strategy. The first was to consider the costs which could be incurred by a range of different groups; the second was to focus not only upon the immediately available information of revenue costs but also to estimate the broader economic effect of a shift in the balance of provision towards community support rather than residential care (the concept of opportunity cost); the third was, where this was appropriate, to discount current costs in order to better reflect the flow of benefits associated with them through time. These principles are summarised below and are discussed in more detail in Netten and Beecham (1993), which examines some of the strategies involved and problems encountered in costing community-based care.

### *A range of different interest groups*

A focus upon shifting the balance of care away from residential and nursing home settings towards enhanced community-based care, in this case mainly by the social services agency, has implications beyond the boundary of just that agency. The individuals receiving services, their families and other agencies will also incur costs and benefits as a consequence of a shift in patterns of provision. In order to provide a realistic broad picture of the impact upon different interest groups, cost estimates were made for a number of different sectors that bear costs. These are: the social services department; the National Health Service; the Department of Social Security; private and not-for-profit agencies providing services; the older person themselves; closely involved carers; and society as a whole. The concept of society as a whole captures the concept of social costs which includes the expenses incurred by older people in their daily living as well as those incurred by their carers in providing support, as well as the costs of all the various forms of service provision that people receive.

In estimating these items of expenditure it was important to ensure that no item was included more than once or included in more than one budget. Similarly, transfer payments were excluded as they have no net effect on costs as a whole. Hence, a pension received from the Department of Social Security would be spent upon the personal consumption of the older person and contributions towards services received and was therefore not treated separately as an item in determining costs to society.

### *Revenue costs and opportunity costs*

The readily available financial reports of agencies usually provide average cost information and the conventions employed in collating these accounts tend to vary. Unsurprisingly therefore, these accounts may not always adequately reflect the consumption of real resources (Sugden and Williams, 1978), or render possible comparisons across accounts.

There are two main cost approaches to be considered: the one commonly employed is revenue cost, the other is the broader economic concept of opportunity cost. Revenue account costs may commonly be broken down into such categories as running costs, maintenance costs, central administrative costs and debt charges. For example, in a residential care home run by a social services department, running costs would include daily expenditure on resources such as heating, lighting and food and the labour costs of employing staff working in the home. Maintenance costs take account of activities such as the replacement of furniture, rewiring and even minor modernisation of the home. Debt charges would represent capital costs arising from repayment on loans used in the construction or major modernisation or extension of the home. Central administrative costs would be those which occur outside the individual unit, concerned with overall administrative services.

As well as capturing the elements of revenue costs, an attempt has been made to ensure that cost estimates are also a reasonable approximation of opportunity cost: that is, based upon an estimate of the value of a resource in terms of benefit forgone by using it in one way rather than in an alternative fashion. Of course in practice such an approach may have to build upon available cost information, but, in making judgements about which capital elements to include, consideration of opportunity costs can be helpful to ensure that different accounts are treated similarly (Knapp, 1984, 1993). An example of this would be the difference in accounting conventions historically employed in different fashions by the National Health Service and local authorities in the inclusion of capital. To provide an estimate of opportunity costs similar capital assumptions were built into the cost estimates.

### Discounting future costs

Costs and any associated benefits may well occur at different times, and in order to make a realistic comparison between alternative forms of service provision it is important to take account of these time lags. For example, provision of intensive community support may promote independent living over a considerable period of time at home, or again an investment now in a wide-ranging assessment process might make it possible for a person to remain at home for a lengthy period, thereby yielding benefit over a period of time considerably greater than that in which the cost is incurred. Both such activities can therefore be described as 'investment goods' the costs of which should be seen as being borne not only at the point at which they were incurred. Therefore, current costs in such situations have been discounted at an appropriate rate, akin to an interest rate, over a suitable time period, in the same way that the construction costs for buildings are frequently discounted over a period of 60 years (Knapp, 1984).

### Unit costs

All cost calculations used figures which applied for the financial year April 1981–March 1982 so as to render them comparable. Since the comparison in the evaluation is between relative cost inputs, the price base is in itself not significant. Notional estimates of current costs may be found in Netten et al. (1999). A consideration of the unit costs relevant to each of the various budgets and the various methods used for estimating costs is presented below.

### Unit costs to the social services department

The social services department unit costs are shown in Table 8.1. In order to estimate the revenue cost of a place in a local authority residential home, figures were used for the most recently built home in the authority, opened three years earlier. The net revenue cost is the gross revenue cost, less the average charges to the older person. In calculating the opportunity cost of a place in residential care, the estimated cost of purchasing the building and land was determined using the method described in the Kent study (Challis and Davies, 1986). The total building and land cost per resident in a 40-bedded home with a 97 per cent occupancy rate worked out at £17,190. Assuming the home would have a 60 years discount period, the weekly capital cost per resident worked out at £17.46 at a discount rate of 5 per cent. These capital costs have been added to the running cost, to give total opportunity costs of £106.47. Where residential and nursing home care was purchased, the contract cost was treated as the unit cost.

Day care provided by the social services department occurred in three settings — day care centres, day care in a residential home and day care supported by volunteers. The cost per service user day in a purpose-built day care centre was £10.32 net revenue cost. Day care in a residential home worked out at £1.55 gross (£1.15 net) per service user day, while day care supported by volunteers came to £2.42 gross (£2.02 net). Although the unit costs of the three types of day care are very different, the type of day care received reflected geographical location within the borough rather than the needs of individuals and higher costs did not necessarily reflect superior quality facilities. It was therefore decided to use a mean unit cost of day care, weighted according to the average number of days of each type consumed by all service users. The ratios of day care usage worked out at day centre — 40 per cent; day care in a residential home — 35 per cent; voluntary day care — 25 per cent. This resulted in the weighted mean costs shown in Table 8.1.

The cost of a care manager's time was calculated assuming a team of two level three social workers and one team leader at senior social worker level who also carried a caseload and was directly responsible to an assistant director. This resulted in an average cost of £5.57 per hour, which included salaries, overheads, clerical support, central administrative costs and travelling expenses. These were lower than for area team social workers due to the lower overhead costs of management.

The cost of an area team social worker's time was estimated assuming a team of eight level three social workers, two senior social workers and one

**Table 8.1**
*Social services department unit costs (price base 1981-82)*

| Type of service | £ |
| --- | --- |
| *Local authority residential home — per week* | |
| Running cost per resident (assuming a 97% occupancy rate) | 82.79 |
| Debt charges | 18.89 |
| Additional central services | 6.27 |
| Total gross revenue cost | 107.95 |
| Total net revenue cost | 81.74 |
| Capital costs discounted at 5% | 17.41 |
| Total opportunity cost (running cost & additional services and central administrative costs & capital costs at 5%) | 106.47 |
| *Day care — per day* | |
| Total gross revenue costs | 5.44 |
| Total net revenue cost | 5.04 |
| Capital costs discounted at 5% | 5.47 |
| Home help — gross cost per hour | 2.29 |
| Home help — net cost per hour | 2.27 |
| Meals-on-wheels — gross cost per meal | 1.32 |
| Meals-on-wheels — net cost per meal | 0.92 |
| Street warden — per week | 0.61 |
| Telephone rental — p.a. | 48.00 |
| Alarm — per lunar month, discounted at 5% | 7.97 |
| ETIS (Emergency Telephone Informative System) — per week | 1.08 |
| Social worker — per hour | 6.00 |

principal social worker, the last three workers having no caseload. The average cost per hour in this case worked out at £6.46. Because care management's organisational costs would become closer to those of area teams through time, it was felt that the hourly cost should not be biased in favour of the scheme. An average of the two hourly rates was therefore used for both care managers and area team social workers, amounting to £6 per hour.

The unit costs of different types of social services department aids were determined from purchasing sources and discounted at a rate of 5 per cent over an appropriate time period.

### Unit costs to the National Health Service

National Health Service unit costs have been summarised in Tables 8.2 and 8.3. They were mainly drawn from the Northern Regional Health Authority Health Service Costs (1982). In-patient, day hospital and day patient opportunity costs

**Table 8.2**
*Unit costs of hospital services including capital element (price base 1981–82)*

| Type of service | £ |
|---|---|
| Acute medical care | 77.22 |
| Mainly acute medical care | 44.17 |
| Long stay geriatric wards and respite beds | 26.32 |
| Psychiatric care | 25.07 |
| Other in-patient days | 58.72 |
| Geriatric/psychiatric day hospital | 18.57 |
| Day patient — acute medical care | 20.17 |

**Table 8.3**
*Unit costs of out-patient and community nursing costs (price base 1981-82)*

| Type of service | £ |
|---|---|
| Medical out-patient appointments | 17.23 |
| Psychiatric out-patient appointments | 10.87 |
| Other out-patient appointments | 3.45 |
| Visits by community SRN, senior nurse or extended nursing service SRN | 3.54 |
| Visits by community SEN or extended nursing service SEN | 2.32 |
| Visits by community nursing auxiliary or extended nursing service auxiliary | 1.81 |
| Night sitting by extended nursing service SRN for 8 hours | 56.64 |

have been determined by adding to the revenue cost a discounted capital component.

This cost component has been worked out using three alternative assumptions regarding buildings (Wright, Cairns and Snell, 1981; Challis and Davies, 1986). The least expensive option is to improve existing buildings without structural alteration. The next possibility is to upgrade buildings with structural alteration. The third and most expensive method is to construct new buildings. For each of these assumptions, the cost was estimated from the values used by Challis and Davies (1986) by means of the Public Sector Building Tender Price Index (Department of the Environment, 1981, 1984). In each case, the capital costs have been determined using a discount rate of 5 per cent. For these scenarios the additional cost element was £0.25, £3.01 and £5.01 respectively. In Table 8.2, National Health Service capital costs have been determined on the assumption that hospital buildings were upgraded, and the same assumption was used for the unit cost of out-patient appointments in Table 8.3.

Community nursing visits were costed according to the type of nurse and were calculated as shown in Table 8.3, each visit being taken to last for half an hour (including travelling). The cost was assumed to be made up of a salary component together with a fixed charge per visit to cover travelling expenses, materials such as dressings and administrative overheads.

### Costs to the social security agency

Information from records provided information on flows of benefits to older people and their carers, which were adjusted for changes in circumstances through time, such as entry to care. These changes in circumstances could have marked effects on flows of benefits and income, such as when one member of an elderly couple was admitted to hospital care.

### Determining the cost to the private and voluntary sector

By far the most important contribution to the private and voluntary sector was from residential homes. It was assumed that the weekly residential charge was on average the cost to social security less the personal allowance of £8.55, which made a net cost of £85.25.

The value of aids supplied by voluntary providers was estimated and discounted over an appropriate period.

### Personal expenditure of the older person

While living in the community, the personal expenditure of the older person was estimated from their gross weekly income using the Family Expenditure Survey (Department of Employment, 1982). The housing component was excluded from this expenditure, as it was taken into account in estimating the housing opportunity cost. This reflected higher personal expenditure according to income and whether or not the person lived alone.

While in institutional care, the personal consumption was taken to be the allowance made for weekly expenditure. This amounted to £5.90 in a local authority residential home or hospital, and £8.55 in a private residential home.

### Costs to informal carers

The additional cost incurred as a result of looking after the older person was estimated from information collected in the interviews with carers. Sometimes this meant a regular amount being spent each week on items such as food and extra heating. In instances where the older person was living in the carer's home and this space might have been used for other purposes, the cost was estimated to include the net loss of income from a potential tenant. Other carers had to give up their employment or reduce their hours of work in order to care and this could result in a substantial loss over the year. As an example of this type of cost, one carer had given up professional employment well before retirement age to care for her mother. She received a pension but at a reduced rate. It was therefore necessary to cost the loss of her future pension and of earnings from employment, less the money received at a reduced level from her pension.

## The value of housing

While an older person is living at home, whether this be owner occupied, council rented or private rented, they occupy housing which would otherwise normally be available, whereas in a care home their accommodation is treated as a cost. In order to determine the resulting cost to society of different care provision, the value of the home was estimated and then discounted at 5 per cent over its lifetime, taken as being 60 years. Housing values were estimated with the assistance of the Nationwide Building Society figures for the relevant period (Nationwide Building Society, 1981). Homes were therefore categorised according to their type and age.

Where an elderly couple were sharing, then the value of their home was divided between them. Moreover, if an older person were living with friends or relatives in accommodation which would not be released when vacated by the older person, then the opportunity cost of that accommodation was taken to be zero.

## Overall cost to society

Total social opportunity cost was determined by summing the relevant component costs considered above. This consisted of the sum of the opportunity costs to the social services department and National Health Service, the social opportunity cost of housing, the costs to the private and voluntary sector and to the older person and their carers.

## The costs of care

The comparison of cost is based upon the 90 matched pairs of cases. There were some interesting variations observed in a number of cost components according to whether or not the older person lived in the inner city area or in the surrounding area, referred to as the outer city area. All costs are therefore shown according to whether the older person was in receipt of the care scheme or was in the comparison group and whether they lived in the inner or outer city area.

All costs have been expressed both as totals over the evaluation year and as costs per week by dividing the annual cost by the number of weeks alive and in the area during the year. This period included time spent in institutional care as well as at home. The cost results for each of the budgets referred to earlier are now considered in turn.

Annual and weekly average costs to the social services department, National Health Service and other parties are shown in Tables 8.4, 8.5, and 8.6 respectively. A summary of the main accounts with statistical tests where appropriate is shown in Table 8.7. The total gross annual and weekly costs to social services, whether calculated as revenue costs or opportunity costs, were lower for those receiving the care scheme, al-though the result was not statistically significant. However, after deducting service user contributions, the net cost to social services was larger for those receiving the care scheme, although this result was also not significant. This was as a result of the much higher contribution paid by those in the comparison group who received substantially more local authority residential care. Changes in charging policies, with relatively higher contributions for those supported in the community, would tend to cause net care scheme costs to be somewhat lower for the department. Gross residential care costs were some ten times higher for the comparison group, and contributed the major part of their cost to the social services department.

Helper fees were the most substantial cost component for the care scheme group and these were substantially higher in the inner city (£19.08 per week) than in the outer city area (£13.14 per week) (p < 0.01). Unsurprisingly, helper expenses were much lower in the inner city, where service users were more geographically concentrated, resulting in lower travelling costs. The care scheme also used substantially more home help support, more than double that for the comparison group (p < 0.01). The time spent by the care managers on each case was some four times greater than that spent by area team social workers with the comparison group when averaged over the time spent alive. However, as the comparison group spent a greater proportion of time in institutional care, the cost per week of social work time spent while the older person was at home was only two and a half times greater for the care scheme. This extra time was important in allowing the care manager to undertake the intensive care management responsibilities. Although those receiving the care scheme received rather more day care, the overall cost was small and the difference between the groups was not statistically significant. Other components of the social services costs were all small although, unsurprisingly, the use of street wardens, social services telephone and alarms was greater for the care scheme group, and aids and adaptations were also loaned more frequently to these older people.

Annual and weekly costs to the National Health Service were somewhat larger for those receiving the care scheme, though the result was not statistically significant. However, costs for the inner city comparison clients were far lower than for the other three groups, and the resulting difference between the inner city and outer city areas was significant (p < 0.05). These inner city comparison group cases received fewer National Health Service resources in spite of their somewhat higher level of dependency, as measured by their capacity to undertake activities of daily living. About half of the National Health Service expenditure was on mainly acute hospital in-patient care, with most of the

**Table 8.4**

*Annual and average weekly cost to the social services department of matched care scheme and comparison cases, broken down according to location (price base 1981-82)*

| Type of cost | Care scheme | | Comparison group | |
|---|---|---|---|---|
| | Annual cost | Weekly cost | Annual cost | Weekly cost |
| *Total SSD gross revenue cost:* | | | | |
| outer city | 1665 | 39.29 | 2260 | 47.71 |
| inner city | 2096 | 43.25 | 1949 | 39.72 |
| *Total SSD net revenue cost:* | | | | |
| outer city | 1609 | 37.69 | 1793 | 37.87 |
| inner city | 2008 | 41.50 | 1535 | 31.34 |
| *Total SSD opportunity cost (5%):* | | | | |
| outer city | 1664 | 39.24 | 2235 | 47.19 |
| inner city | 2094 | 43.21 | 1926 | 39.28 |
| *Residential care gross revenue cost:* | | | | |
| outer city | 115 | 3.98 | 1850 | 38.95 |
| inner city | 175 | 3.46 | 1639 | 33.08 |
| *Residential care net revenue cost:* | | | | |
| outer city | 87 | 3.01 | 1402 | 29.50 |
| inner city | 133 | 2.62 | 1241 | 25.06 |
| *Day care mix net revenue cost:* | | | | |
| outer city | 46 | 0.95 | 31 | 0.59 |
| inner city | 57 | 1.10 | 21 | 0.56 |
| *Care scheme day care:* | | | | |
| outer city | 74 | 1.43 | - | - |
| inner city | 59 | 1.13 | - | - |
| *Care scheme helper — fees:* | | | | |
| outer city | 599 | 13.14 | - | - |
| inner city | 938 | 19.08 | - | - |
| *Care scheme helper — expenses:* | | | | |
| outer city | 59 | 1.24 | - | - |
| inner city | 43 | 0.91 | - | - |
| *Home help net cost:* | | | | |
| outer city | 393 | 9.21 | 182 | 4.11 |
| inner city | 319 | 6.35 | 150 | 3.08 |
| *Meals-on-wheels net cost:* | | | | |
| outer city | 48 | 1.09 | 32 | 0.72 |
| inner city | 86 | 1.76 | 31 | 0.67 |
| *Care scheme social work:* | | | | |
| outer city | 294 | 7.44 | - | - |
| inner city | 347 | 8.02 | - | - |
| *Area team social work:* | | | | |
| outer city | - | - | 145 | 2.91 |
| inner city | - | - | 90 | 1.94 |

**Table 8.5**

*Annual and average weekly costs to the National Health Service of matched care scheme and comparison cases, broken down according to location (price base 1981-82)*

| Type of cost | Care scheme | | Comparison group | |
|---|---|---|---|---|
| | Annual cost | Weekly cost | Annual cost | Weekly cost |
| Total NHS revenue cost: | | | | |
| outer city | 1706 | 48.09 | 1481 | 39.22 |
| inner city | 1408 | 40.47 | 454 | 11.66 |
| Total NHS opportunity cost (5%): | | | | |
| outer city | 1798 | 50.80 | 1588 | 42.04 |
| inner city | 1505 | 43.09 | 483 | 12.34 |
| Acute hospital revenue cost: | | | | |
| outer city | 660 | 18.26 | 373 | 7.18 |
| inner city | 281 | 11.57 | 36 | 2.30 |
| Acute hospital opportunity cost (5%): | | | | |
| outer city | 687 | 19.00 | 388 | 7.47 |
| inner city | 292 | 12.04 | 37 | 2.39 |
| Mainly acute hospital revenue cost: | | | | |
| outer city | 651 | 20.29 | 765 | 25.13 |
| inner city | 741 | 21.04 | 253 | 5.73 |
| Mainly acute hospital opportunity cost (5%): | | | | |
| outer city | 698 | 21.77 | 821 | 26.96 |
| inner city | 795 | 22.58 | 272 | 6.14 |
| Long stay geriatric hospital revenue cost: | | | | |
| outer city | 67 | 2.38 | 55 | 1.06 |
| inner city | 22 | 0.49 | 35 | 0.68 |
| Long stay geriatric hospital opportunity cost (5%): | | | | |
| outer city | 75 | 2.69 | 62 | 1.20 |
| inner city | 25 | 0.55 | 40 | 0.77 |
| Respite bed revenue cost: | | | | |
| outer city | 30 | 0.58 | 0 | 0.00 |
| inner city | 11 | 0.21 | 6 | 0.12 |
| Respite bed opportunity cost (5%): | | | | |
| outer city | 34 | 0.65 | 0 | 0.00 |
| inner city | 12 | 0.24 | 7 | 0.14 |
| Psychiatric hospital revenue cost: | | | | |
| outer city | 13 | 0.26 | 204 | 0.14 |
| inner city | 182 | 3.50 | 17 | 0.33 |
| Psychiatric hospital opportunity cost (5%): | | | | |
| outer city | 15 | 0.29 | 232 | 4.46 |
| inner city | 207 | 3.98 | 20 | 0.37 |

**Table 8.5 (continued)**

| Type of cost | Care scheme | | Comparison group | |
|---|---|---|---|---|
| | Annual cost | Weekly cost | Annual cost | Weekly cost |
| *Geriatric day hospital revenue cost:* | | | | |
| outer city | 2 | 0.06 | 0 | 0.00 |
| inner city | 10 | 0.20 | 6 | 0.12 |
| *Geriatric day hospital opportunity cost (5%):* | | | | |
| outer city | 2 | 0.07 | 0 | 0.00 |
| inner city | 12 | 0.23 | 7 | 0.14 |
| *Psychiatric day hospital revenue cost:* | | | | |
| outer city | 16 | 0.30 | 0 | 0.00 |
| inner city | 0 | 0.00 | 0 | 0.00 |
| *Psychiatric day hospital opportuntiy cost (5%):* | | | | |
| outer city | 19 | 0.36 | 0 | 0.00 |
| inner city | 0 | 0.00 | 0 | 0.00 |
| *Community nursing visits:* | | | | |
| outer city | 252 | 5.64 | 47 | 1.19 |
| inner city | 150 | 3.22 | 86 | 2.03 |

remainder coming from acute hospital care, and it was these resources which were so much lower for those in the comparison group in the inner city area. Other types of hospital in-patient care were small and geriatric and psychiatric day hospital care were little used.The other important contribution to National Health Service costs was from community nursing. This was mainly from RGN visits which were much more frequent for the care scheme group (p < 0.01), especially in the outer city area. This probably indicates closer working between the care scheme and community nursing teams in this area, with more frequent assessment and review visits.

Table 8.6 shows costs to other parties. Practically all costs within the private and voluntary sector resulted from provision of places in residential homes. The only other cost came from the use of aids on loan from voluntary agencies. The total cost was only important for those in the comparison group living in the inner city, for whom it averaged £2.60 per week. The weekly personal consumption of older people in the comparison group worked out at substantially less than for those receiving the care scheme (p < 0.01). This was a result of those in the comparison group spending considerably longer in institutional care, where personal expenditure was limited to a weekly allowance. Costs to carers averaged out at a relatively small amount, between £1 and £2 per week for each of the groups. Although this was higher in the outer city area, the effect was not significant. It would therefore appear that the main cost to the carers studied was to their psychological well-being and their leisure time,

Table 8.6

*Annual and average weekly costs to other budgets of matched care schemes and comparison cases, according to location (price base 1981-82)*

| Type of cost | Care scheme | | Comparison group | |
|---|---|---|---|---|
| | Annual cost | Weekly cost | Annual cost | Weekly Cost |
| Private and voluntary sector: | | | | |
| outer city | 3 | 0.06 | 0 | 0.00 |
| inner city | 3 | 0.05 | 132 | 2.60 |
| Personal consumption of older person excluding housing: | | | | |
| outer city | 1020 | 23.18 | 794 | 16.96 |
| inner city | 1116 | 23.29 | 848 | 18.57 |
| Informal carers: | | | | |
| outer city | 92 | 1.98 | 72 | 1.54 |
| inner city | 42 | 1.11 | 59 | 1.20 |
| Housing opportunity cost (5%): | | | | |
| outer city | 643 | 15.63 | 515 | 11.38 |
| inner city | 573 | 12.19 | 398 | 9.05 |
| Social Security: | | | | |
| outer city | 1667 | 38.21 | 1775 | 38.55 |
| inner city | 1919 | 39.88 | 1751 | 37.87 |

rather than a financial one. However, were a broader approach to the costing of carers' time to be used, then carer costs would have appeared substantial. As was shown in Chapter 7 however, this would have been lower for the care scheme group. The weekly housing opportunity cost worked out rather more for those receiving the care scheme (p < 0.01). This was attributable to their spending a greater amount of time in the community. The average cost to the social security agency showed very little variation between the groups. The average time spent at home, including periods of short-term or respite care varied considerably between the groups, with those receiving the care scheme remaining at home longer (p < 0.01). Thus, in the outer city area the care scheme group were at home for 42 weeks and the comparison group for 32 weeks; and in the inner city area for 45 and 34 weeks respectively.

A summary of the main cost accounts is shown in Table 8.7. In comparing average costs between care scheme and comparison groups analysis of variance was used, to determine whether the difference between average values could have occurred simply by chance. These differences could be between either the care scheme and comparison groups or the inner city and outer city groups. The probability that any relationship, or 'interaction', between the joint influences of receiving the care scheme and living in the inner city could have happened by chance was also estimated in the analysis. The meaning of interaction may be illustrated by a simple example. Suppose a particular

**Table 8.7**
*Annual and average weekly costs to main budgets of matched care scheme and comparison cases, according to location (price base 1981-82)*

| Cost budget | £ | | Tests | |
|---|---|---|---|---|
| | Care scheme | Comparison group | Scheme v Comparison | Outer v inner city |
| **Annual Costs** | | | | |
| *Total SSD gross revenue cost:* | | | | |
| outer city | 1665 | 2260 | ns | ns |
| inner city | 2096 | 1949 | | |
| *Total SSD net revenue cost:* | | | | |
| outer city | 1609 | 1793 | ns | ns |
| inner city | 2008 | 1535 | | |
| *Total SSD opportunity cost (5%):* | | | | |
| outer city | 1664 | 2235 | ns | ns |
| inner city | 2094 | 1926 | | |
| *Total NHS opportunity cost (5%):* | | | | |
| outer city | 1798 | 1588 | ns | <0.05 |
| inner city | 1505 | 483 | | |
| *Total opp. cost to SSD and NHS (5%):* | | | | |
| outer city | 3461 | 3823 | ns* | ns |
| inner city | 3599 | 2409 | | |
| *Social opportunity cost (5%):* | | | | |
| outer city | 5220 | 5203 | ns | ns |
| inner city | 5333 | 3847 | | |
| **Average Weekly Costs** | | | | |
| *Total SSD gross revenue cost:* | 39.29 | 47.71 | ns | ns |
| outer city | 43.25 | 39.72 | | |
| inner city | | | | |
| *Total SSD net revenue cost:* | 37.69 | 37.87 | ns | ns |
| outer city | 41.50 | 31.34 | | |
| inner city | | | | |
| *Total SSD opportunity cost (5%):* | 39.24 | 47.19 | ns | ns |
| outer city | 43.21 | 39.28 | | |
| inner city | | | | |
| *Total NHS opportunity cost (5%):* | 50.80 | 42.04 | ns | <0.05 |
| outer city | 43.09 | 12.34 | | |
| inner city | | | | |
| *Total opp. cost to SSD and NHS (5%):* | | | | |
| outer city | 90.04 | 89.23 | ns* | <0.01 |
| inner city | 86.29 | 51.62 | | |
| *Social opportunity cost (5%):* | | | | |
| outer city | 130.90 | 119.10 | <0.05 | <0.01 |
| inner city | 122.96 | 83.05 | | |

ns = not significant.
* = significant interaction effect.

average cost to be small for care scheme cases in the outer area and for comparison cases in the inner city area but large otherwise. It is then possible for there to be no significant difference between averages for care scheme and comparison cases or outer and inner city cases, and yet for significant interaction to occur. In comparing the significance of differences in cost between the groups the stability of the estimates were further tested by including indicators of ADL (Activities of Daily Living) and psychological well-being as covariates in the analysis of variance.

It was found that the group of care scheme cases living in the outer area lived on average somewhat less long (42.5 weeks) than the comparison cases in that area (46.3 weeks), or the care scheme and comparison clients in the inner city area (47.2 weeks and 46.6 weeks respectively). Although the difference is not statistically significant, it makes annual costs appear relatively smaller for care scheme cases outside the inner city than would otherwise be the case. Examination of the pattern of care of cases who did not survive for the full year suggested that those individuals tended to be more needy and have higher costs. However, those who survived for a short while were relatively few in number and there was no evidence to suggest that such short care episodes distorted the overall pattern of costs.

Table 8.7 shows the total annual and weekly costs to the main budgets. Costs to social services and the National Health Service taken together are also included. With capital costs discounted at 5 per cent, the combined weekly opportunity cost to these two budgets was very similar, in the range £86–£90, for three of the groups, but inner city comparison cases cost substantially less, £52, due to considerably lower use of National Health Service resources. This resulted in inner city cases being significantly less costly ($p < 0.01$), although the extra cost of the care scheme over comparison cases was not significant.

At a discount rate of 5 per cent, the weekly cost to society worked out as somewhat greater for care scheme cases ($p < 0.05$). This effect was not evident for annual costs and is explained by the small differences in survival rates noted earlier.

### Summary of the costs of care

The gross weekly opportunity cost to the social services department in Gateshead appeared to be very similar for both the care scheme and standard provision. However, the authority charging policy at that time required the older person to pay a much larger proportion of the cost of residential care than of domiciliary services. As a result of those in the comparison group spending more time in residential care, their costs to the social services department appeared lower than for the care scheme group, although the difference was still not significant.

The weekly opportunity cost to the National Health Service emerged as not significantly different between the care scheme and standard provision.

However, the cost of standard provision in the inner city was a great deal lower (at £12.34 per week) than that in the outer area (£42.04) (p < 0.05). However, the higher cost of those receiving the care scheme in this area may be in part a result of the care managers' ability to successfully negotiate resources that would otherwise not have been provided. The extra cost of the care managers' cases might therefore be seen as compensation for an otherwise rather low National Health Service provision.

The overall cost to society was significantly greater on a weekly basis for care managers' cases. However most of the difference appeared to be as a result of the lower National Health Service resources received by the comparison group in the inner city. In the outer area the additional cost to society for the care scheme group was much smaller. The reduced costs to the comparison group of personal consumption and housing as a result of the larger proportion of time spent in institutional care also contributed to the difference in total social costs.

Thus, in Table 8.7 most costs appeared to be no higher for care scheme cases than for those in the comparison group, a result which should be set against the relative success of the scheme in improving quality of life and in enabling older people to remain for longer in their own homes.

## Costs and outcomes

In the early part of this chapter the average costs of the care scheme to different budgets were determined, and compared with those for the matched comparison group who were receiving standard care provision. The change in different measures of quality of life was investigated in Chapter 6 for the older people, and in Chapter 7 for the carers, and a comparison made between the groups receiving the care scheme and standard provision. Of course, average cost comparisons conceal variations and further analysis was required to understand the factors that appeared to systematically influence cost. Hence, an analysis of variation may explain at least as much as a comparison of aggregates, as well as permitting a degree of compensation for any differences between groups (Challis and Darton, 1990). The remainder of this chapter examines the relationship between costs, need characteristics and changes in quality of life. This includes estimates of the average cost of improving aspects of quality of life by a given amount for both the care scheme and comparison groups, thereby providing further evidence about their relative effectiveness and efficiency.

As in previous studies, the 'production of welfare' approach was adopted (Challis et al., 1995), in which the changes in quality of life and well-being during the year (outcomes) are seen as depending on both the older person's initial physical and mental states and circumstances (quasi-inputs or need indicators) and the resources consumed during the year (costs). The underlying premise of this approach is that costs, and therefore patterns of service, are determined by client need characteristics, social environment and social support, and the outcomes of care. Much of the complexity involved in comprehending the care process arises from the ways in which these cost factors (services) and need characteristics interact (Challis and Darton, 1990).

Quasi inputs or need characteristics covered seven areas: health and dependency, social support, personality and attitudes to help, personal characteristics and living environment, initial levels of well-being, health status and carer stress. Six outcome indicators were identified. The first was the length of survival time over one year measured in weeks. Three were mainly relevant to social care: quality of care, subjective well-being and carer malaise or stress. Two were mainly relevant to health care: general health and activities of daily living. Subjective well-being was measured using the Philadelphia Geriatric Center Morale Scale (Lawton, 1972). Quality of care was measured by aggregating the measures of need shortfall in four areas: personal care, rising and retiring, daily and weekly household care (Challis and Davies, 1986). Malaise was measured using the malaise scale (Rutter et al., 1970). General health was made up of the sum of the number of subjective and symptomatic health items present and activities of daily living was measured as the sum of the six key activities of daily living (Katz et al., 1963). Except for survival, each outcome indicator was standardised so that the difference between first and second assessments was expressed as a percentage improvement or decline in well-being.

This list of the predictor variables from which these outcomes and need indicators were selected is shown in Box 8.1. Multiple regression analysis was used to estimate the relationship between these and different aspects of cost. When predictor variables were missing, the average for the group as a whole was used. This included circumstances such as when follow-up material was missing for people who had died within the year. The corresponding mean values were then used to determine the outputs, as in other studies (Challis et al., 1995), since exclusion of such cases might yield a more partial and biased analysis.

## Patterns of variation in costs

In these analyses, four sets of cost equations are presented. The first two represent costs to each of the two main agencies, health and social services, and the second two costs to the agencies combined and costs to society. The cost measures, which are the dependent variables in this analysis, are the annual total cost for each of the accounts cited. The equations are shown in Tables 8.8 to 8.15.

**Box 8.1**
*Variables used in predicting costs*

| DOMAIN/VARIABLE | VARIABLE FORM |
|---|---|
| **Health and dependency** | |
| Arthritis | None, moderate, severe |
| Eyesight difficulties | None, moderate, severe |
| Hearing difficulties | None, moderate, severe |
| Giddiness | None, moderate, severe |
| Breathlessness | None, moderate, severe |
| Risk of falling | None, moderate, severe |
| Incontinence of urine | None, occasional, frequent |
| Incontinence of faeces | None, occasional, frequent |
| Dependency states | Dependency groups 1,2,3,4 |
| Confusion/disorientation | Score of 2 or more on items about behaviour, appearance, memory, range 0-9 |
| Depressed mood | None, mild, moderate, severe |
| Felt capacity to cope | Sum of responses to 4 questions about capacity to cope with daily living, range 4-16 |
| Loneliness | Sum of responses to 2 questions about loneliness and dissatisfaction, range 0-6 |
| Anxiety | None, mild, moderate, severe |

| | |
|---|---|
| **Social support** | |
| All formal/informal care | Total weekly social contacts |
| Presence of informal carer | Yes or no |
| Living with spouse | Yes or no |
| Living with relatives | Yes or no |
| Support from children | Number of weekly social contacts |
| Support from relatives | Number of weekly social contacts |
| Support from neighbours/friends | Number of weekly social contacts |
| Support from informal carer | Presence or absence |
| Whether has confidant(e) | Presence or absence |

| | |
|---|---|
| **Personality and attitudes to help** | |
| Hostile–rejecting | Characteristic present or absent |
| Passive–dependent | Characteristic present or absent |
| Dependent–demanding | Characteristic present or absent |

| | |
|---|---|
| **Personal characteristics and living environment** | |
| Location | Inner city or outer city |
| Housing problems | Number of identified problems |
| Overall suitability of housing | Suitable, unsuitable, detrimental |
| Dissatisfaction with housing | Number of reasons |
| Age | Years |
| Gender | Male or female |
| Whether retired to area | Yes or no |
| Recent bereavement | Yes or no |

| Box 8.1 (continued) |
| --- |

| DOMAIN/VARIABLE | VARIABLE FORM |
| --- | --- |
| **Initial level of well-being** | |
| Quality of care | Sum of measures of need shortfall — rising/ retiring, personal care, daily and weekly housework |
| Subjective well-being | Philadelphia Geriatric Center Score, range 0-17 |
| **Initial health status** | |
| General health | Sum of subjective level of ill health and individual health items, range 1-18 |
| Activities of daily living | Sum of individual activities requiring help, range 0-6 |
| **Initial carer stress** | |
| Malaise score | A Malaise score of 7 or more, range 0-24 |
| **Outcomes** | |
| Quality of care | Per cent improvement or decline |
| Subjective well-being | Per cent improvement or decline |
| Survival | Weeks survived |
| General Health | Per cent improvement or decline |
| Activities of daily living | Per cent improvement or decline |
| Malaise | Per cent improvement or decline |

**Table 8.8**

*Cost of outcomes to the social services department for the care scheme group, £, at 1981 prices*

| Variable | Cost effect £ | p value |
| --- | --- | --- |
| **Need indicators** | | |
| *Health and dependency* | | |
| Loneliness | 115.21 | 0.013 |
| *Social support* | | |
| Living with family | -931.23 | <0.001 |
| **Outcomes** | | |
| (Quality of care)$^2$, $Q^2$ | 0.07 | <0.001 |
| (Subjective well-being)$^2$, $M^2$ | 0.02 | 0.040 |
| (Subjective well-being)(Quality of care), MQ | -0.07 | <0.001 |
| Survival (weeks) | 40.48 | <0.001 |
| Constant | -1186.91 | <0.001 |

$F = 32.9$
p value $<0.001$
$R^2 = 0.70$
Adj. $R^2 = 0.68$

**Table 8.9**
*Cost of outcomes to the social services department for the comparison group, £,
at 1981 prices*

| Variable | Cost effect £ | p value |
|---|---|---|
| **Need indicators** | | |
| *Health and dependency* | | |
| Eyesight difficulties | -306.17 | 0.048 |
| Arthritis | -288.61 | 0.035 |
| *Personality and attitude to help* | | |
| Hostile-rejecting attitude | -1622.57 | 0.004 |
| *Other factors* | | |
| Whether living in inner city | -407.23 | 0.091 |
| **Outcomes** | | |
| (Quality of care)$^2$, $Q^2$ | 0.12 | <0.001 |
| (Subjective well-being)(Quality of care), MQ | -0.05 | 0.002 |
| Survival (weeks) | 27.26 | 0.006 |
| Constant | -44.80 | 0.957 |

F = 12.4
p value <0.001
$R^2$ = 0.58
Adj. $R^2$ = 0.54

## The cost to the social services department

The equations are shown in Tables 8.8 and 8.9 for the care scheme and comparison group respectively. It was possible to obtain a reasonably accurate prediction of the cost to social services of standard provision (adjusted $R^2$ = 0.54),
and a still better fit for the care scheme (adjusted $R^2$ = 0.68). In the case of standard provision the main contribution towards high cost was time spent in residential care, which accounted for 77 per cent of expenditure.

*Health and dependency* A noteworthy feature for each group was that none of
the aspects of physical disability or ill-health appeared to be associated with increased cost to the social services department. The presence of eyesight difficulties in the comparison group resulted in a smaller predicted annual cost.
Although these cases had a shorter life expectancy, this did not lead to a higher
uptake of residential care. They were more likely to either remain at home or
die at home and were more often living with their family, which reduced cost.
Comparison cases suffering from arthritis were also less likely to be admitted to
a residential home and were therefore less costly. Amongst the care scheme
group loneliness was responsible for a small additional cost, mainly through
additional expenditure on day care for those on their own.

*Social support* In the care scheme group those living with family cost significantly less over the year as a result of the substantial number of tasks which carers normally undertook, hence reducing the level of provision by social services.

*Personality and attitudes to help* Those older people with a more hostile or rejecting attitude to help might either have refused services offered or caused these services to regularly break down, resulting in a reduction in cost. The fact that this reduction was only evident in standard provision points to the ability of the scheme to obtain access in difficult circumstances normally beyond the scope of standard provision, with care managers having time and flexible resources to ensure such individuals did in fact receive help.

*Physical environment and other factors* Inner city cases were less costly in standard provision reflecting a lower level of resources overall. However this difference did not emerge in the care scheme, reflecting the ability of the scheme to offer a more equitable uniform level of service by having the flexibility to fill gaps in the availability of conventional services. Moreover, by supporting the majority of older people at home over the evaluation year, area differences in the availability of residential care had little effect on costs.

*Outcomes* For the care scheme group the cost of an increase in either subjective well-being (M) or quality of care (Q) contains a quadratic term. This indicates increasingly higher costs of obtaining higher improvements in either of these indicators, in short diminishing returns of extra services once a certain level of well-being was achieved. The negative joint term between subjective well-being and quality of care (MQ) illustrates the effect of joint supply in achieving improvements in these two outputs. It suggests that services designed to improve quality of care could simultaneously have an effect in improving subjective well-being. Subjective well-being was directly associated with costs in the care scheme, indicating that interventions were directly focused upon this area of need, as well as in association with meeting practical care needs. However, this was not the case for standard provision, where the presence of the joint term between quality of care and subjective well-being suggests that interventions were more likely to impact upon older people's subjective well-being through meeting practical care needs.

### The cost to the National Health Service

Tables 8.10 and 8.11 show costs to the National Health Service for the care scheme and comparison group respectively. Unsurprisingly, it was only possible to predict a relatively small proportion of the variation in cost to the National Health Service using the variables available, 36 per cent for the care scheme and 26 per cent for standard provision. Without more detailed clinical

UNIVERSITY OF WINCHESTER
LIBRARY

**Table 8.10**
*Cost of outcomes to the National Health Service for the care scheme group, £, at 1981 prices*

| Variable | Cost effect £ | p value |
|---|---|---|
| **Need indicators** | | |
| *Health and dependency* | | |
| Breathlessness | 646.52 | 0.032 |
| Risk of falling | 1570.37 | <0.001 |
| Anxiety | 574.63 | 0.078 |
| Confusion/disorientation | 1002.43 | 0.049 |
| *Personality and attitude to help* | | |
| Passive-dependent attitude | 4846.05 | <0.001 |
| **Outcomes** | | |
| (General health)$^2$, $G^2$ | -0.15 | <0.001 |
| Improvement in carer Malaise to below | | |
| threshold stress level | 14.12 | 0.030 |
| Constant | -2653.02 | 0.036 |
| F = 8.1 | | |
| p value <0.001 | | |
| $R^2$ = 0.41 | | |
| Adj. $R^2$ = 0.36 | | |

information available at the time of assessment it would not be expected to predict, with any accuracy, which cases would incur for example the very high costs of acute hospital in-patient treatment.

*Health and dependency* In both groups, those cases with a higher initial level of anxiety incurred higher cost, mainly through a greater use of hospital in-patient care, reflecting an association of anxiety with poor health. Risk of falling, confusion/disorientation and breathlessness amongst care scheme cases were all associated with increased cost. Both risk of falling and breathlessness, the latter associated with chest disease, led to more time being spent in acute hospital settings and a greater use of community nursing care. Those with confusional states spent longer in both psychiatric and acute hospitals. Certainly care managers made considerable effort to access appropriate health care for these cases. For those receiving standard provision, these three need categories did not generally receive any additional hospital or community nursing care. This appeared to be particularly so in the inner city areas.

*Social support* People receiving standard provision who lived with a spouse consumed considerably more National Health Service resources, reflecting the

**Table 8.11**
*Cost of outcomes to the National Health Service for the comparison group, £, at 1981 prices*

| Variable | Cost effect £ | p value |
|---|---|---|
| **Need indicators** | | |
| *Health and dependency* | | |
|   Anxiety | 492.52 | 0.077 |
| *Social support* | | |
|   Lives with spouse | 2454.39 | 0.003 |
| *Personality and attitude to help* | | |
|   Passive-dependent attitude | 1840.17 | 0.070 |
| *Other factors* | | |
|   Gender: whether female | -2094.04 | 0.004 |
|   Whether living in inner city | -1143.65 | 0.018 |
| *Initial health status* | | |
|   Activities of daily living score | 228.83 | 0.099 |
| **Outcomes** | | |
| General Health, G | 14.17 | 0.087 |
| (Activities of daily living)x(General health), AG | -0.14 | 0.003 |
| Constant | 4657.32 | 0.011 |

$F = 4.9$
p value $<0.001$
$R^2 = 0.32$
Adj. $R^2 = 0.26$

needs of a few very frail individuals who received considerable amounts of in-patient care. No such effect was visible for the care scheme group.

*Personality and attitudes to help* In each group, cases with a passive-dependent attitude to help were substantially more expensive as expected, these cases being likely either to receive or accept more domiciliary nursing support, or a higher level of hospital care when this was suggested by professionals.

*Other factors* The gender of the older person was an important determinant of the cost of standard provision, older men having higher costs due, in this instance, to their greater use of acute hospital care. Older people receiving standard provision located in the inner city received substantially fewer National Health Service resources (amounting to £1144 less per annum) than those in the outer city area. This reflects the comparison of the costs of matched groups, namely that National Health Service resource allocation in standard provision was considerably less in the inner city area. In the care scheme, the actions of the care managers appeared to compensate for this, and location did not appear to affect the level of National Health Service cost.

*Initial health status* Unsurprisingly, cases receiving standard provision with a higher initial ADL score, a measure of dependency, incurred higher National Health Service expenditure.

*Outcomes* In standard provision, a positive general health term and a stronger negative product term between improvements in general health (G) and ADL score (A) were the only outputs. Increased expenditure was usually associated with a deterioration in both functional status and general health. A negative general health effect was observed for care scheme cases. These findings suggest that the relationship between health status changes and long-term care services is, generally as would be expected, one where changes in health status lead to changes in service allocations rather than vice versa.

For care scheme cases a clear relationship emerged between increased National Health Service expenditure and improvement in the Malaise score of a carer to a level of stress below the threshold. This reflected the relief of carer stress associated with the admission of the older person into long-stay hospital care and provision of community nursing. This reflects the findings of Levin et al. (1989) for the confused elderly and their families.

### The cost to society

The equations for costs to society are shown as Tables 8.12 and 8.13. It was possible to obtain a cost equation with a reasonably good fit for the care scheme group (adj. $R^2 = 0.53$), with less of the cost variation accounted for in the comparison group (adj. $R^2 = 0.45$).

*Health and dependency* As was the case with National Health Service costs, anxiety was again associated with higher cost in standard provision through a link with poor health and the greater use of hospital in-patient beds. Those in the care scheme group who saw themselves able to cope were less costly.

*Social support* In both groups, the presence of an informal carer was associated with an increased overall cost to society, though this effect was stronger for care scheme cases, reflecting the higher levels of support given to carers, and the higher dependency of these cases. Amongst care scheme cases, as well as any increase in cost associated with the presence of an informal carer was a smaller reduction in cost when the older person was supported by neighbours or friends. For cases receiving standard provision, costs were higher when the older person was living with a spouse, which as before was associated with more in-patient care.

**Table 8.12**
*Cost of outcomes to society for the care scheme group, £, at 1981 prices*

| Variable | Cost effect £ | p value |
|---|---|---|
| **Need indicators** | | |
| *Health and dependency* | | |
| Felt capacity to cope | -632.03 | 0.009 |
| *Social support* | | |
| Contact with neighbours | -73.19 | 0.055 |
| Presence of an informal carer | 1211.75 | 0.009 |
| *Personality and attitude to help* | | |
| Passive-dependent attitude | 3845.50 | <0.001 |
| *Other factors* | | |
| Gender: whether female | 1126.07 | 0.093 |
| *Initial level of well-being* | | |
| Subjective well-being | -121.61 | 0.044 |
| *Initial health status* | | |
| General health problem score | 155.84 | 0.031 |
| **Outcomes** | | |
| Quality of care, Q | -78.85 | <0.001 |
| (Quality of care)$^2$, Q$^2$ | 0.22 | 0.009 |
| (Subjective well-being)$^2$, M$^2$ | -0.15 | <0.001 |
| (Subjective well-being)x(Quality of care), MQ | 0.18 | 0.013 |
| Survival (weeks) | 95.44 | <0.001 |
| Constant | 8967.03 | 0.004 |

F = 8.8
p value <0.001
$R^2$ = 0.60
Adj. $R^2$ = 0.53

*Personality and attitudes to help* Cases with a passive-dependent attitude to help were, as observed for National Health Service costs, a source of higher social cost in both groups. For such cases receiving standard provision periods in long-term residential care or geriatric hospital were more frequent. Those receiving the care scheme, although unlikely to enter long-term institutional care, had more episodes of acute hospital care.

*Physical environment and other factors* As was the case for National Health Service costs, males receiving standard provision had higher costs than females. However, for those in receipt of the care scheme, costs were greater for females, because they lived proportionately longer. Recent bereavement was also associated with lower cost for standard provision as a result of fewer admissions to

**Table 8.13**
*Cost of outcomes to society for the comparison group, £, at 1981 prices*

| Variable | Cost effect £ | p value |
|---|---|---|
| ***Need indicators*** | | |
| *Health and dependency* | | |
| Anxiety | 617.49 | 0.024 |
| *Social support* | | |
| Lives with spouse | 2025.80 | 0.008 |
| Presence of an informal carer | 818.69 | 0.095 |
| *Personality and attitude to help* | | |
| Passive-dependent attitude | 1543.26 | 0.102 |
| *Other factors* | | |
| Gender: whether female | -2263.19 | 0.001 |
| Bereavement during last year | -1172.69 | 0.015 |
| Whether living in inner city | -1501.37 | 0.001 |
| ***Outcomes*** | | |
| Quality of care, Q | 13.09 | 0.007 |
| Survival (weeks) | 89.27 | <0.001 |
| Constant | 3788.65 | 0.050 |

$F = 9.0$
p value $<0.001$
$R^2 = 0.50$
Adj. $R^2 = 0.45$

institutional care. As was the case for National Health Service expenditure, costs were significantly lower in the inner city area for standard provision.

*Initial health status* Care scheme cases in poor health were more likely to incur higher costs as might be expected. In the same vein, higher levels of subjective well-being were associated with lower costs.

*Outcomes* In considering the relationship between outputs and total social cost, outputs were restricted to those involving quality of care (Q) and subjective well-being (M), as these were most readily amenable to influence by the implementation of the care scheme. The relationship between health status and services discussed earlier in the National Health Service analyses appeared to confirm this. For those receiving standard provision, a simple relationship between cost and improvement in quality of care emerged, whilst subjective well-being did not prove to be associated with cost. However, for the care scheme group, the relationship was more complex. Improvements in subjective well-being were associated with lower costs, and this, coupled with the positive interaction term (MQ) indicated that the two outcomes were provided both jointly and individually in relation to levels of service input. Conversely, in standard provision, the lack of relationship between subjective well-being and cost, could indicate the focus of services upon meeting practical care needs alone, rather than the wider needs of the older person.

## Cost to agencies

The equations for costs to the two main agencies, health and social services, are shown as Tables 8.14 and 8.15. As costs to the social services department and National Health Service when taken separately present only a partial picture of the deployment of resources, the relationship between costs and outputs was also examined when expenditure to these agencies was combined. Moreover, decisions regarding the allocation of cases between local authority and private residential care depended more on the availability of a place than on their relative merits. It was therefore decided, in calculating the cost to agencies, that private residential care should be included as though it were local authority residential care. This would be consistent with the current methods of funding community care. The main difference with total social cost is the omission of

**Table 8.14**
*Cost of outcomes to the social services department and National Health Service combined for the care scheme group, £, at 1981 prices*

| Variable | Cost effect £ | p value |
|---|---|---|
| **Need indicators** | | |
| *Health and dependency* | | |
|   Risk of falling | 1081.97 | 0.003 |
|   Felt capacity of cope | -589.97 | 0.020 |
| *Personality and attitude to help* | | |
|   Passive-dependent attitude | 4408.73 | <0.001 |
| **Outcomes** | | |
| (Subjective well-being)$^2$, $M^2$ | -0.05 | 0.034 |
| Improvement in carer Malaise from critical stress | | |
|   to non-critical | 18.17 | 0.013 |
| Survival (weeks) | 55.33 | <0.001 |
| Constant | 3225.47 | 0.160 |
| $F = 6.9$ | | |
| p value $<0.001$ | | |
| $R^2 = 0.40$ | | |
| Adj. $R^2 = 0.35$ | | |

Cost totals are net opportunity costs, discounted at 5 per cent. Days spent in private residential care are treated as though they were extra days in a local authority residential home.

**Table 8.15**

*Cost of outcomes to the social services department and National Health Service combined for the comparison group, £, at 1981 prices*

| Variable | Cost effect £ | p value |
|---|---|---|
| **Quasi-inputs** | | |
| *Health and dependency* | | |
| Anxiety | 708.15 | 0.014 |
| *Social support* | | |
| Lives with spouse | 2469.83 | 0.003 |
| *Personality and attitude to help* | | |
| Passive-dependent attitude | 1818.26 | 0.072 |
| *Other factors* | | |
| Gender: whether female | -2219.02 | 0.003 |
| Bereavement during the past year | -1245.28 | 0.014 |
| Whether living in inner city | -1427.52 | 0.003 |
| **Outcomes** | | |
| (Quality of care)$^2$, $Q^2$ | 0.07 | 0.004 |
| Survival (weeks) | 38.72 | 0.037 |
| Constant | 4940.46 | 0.012 |
| $F = 7.82$ | | |
| p value $<0.001$ | | |
| $R^2 = 0.43$ | | |
| Adj. $R^2 = 0.38$ | | |

Cost totals are net opportunity costs, discounted at 5 per cent. Days spent in private residential care are treated as though they were extra days in a local authority residential home.

the social cost of housing, which did not play a central part in the care process, and the non-inclusion of costs borne by carers. Although the equation for standard provision was fairly similar to the corresponding one for costs to society, the care scheme equation showed some important differences.

*Health and dependency* The results were similar to those for total social cost, except that risk of falling now appeared as a determinant of cost for care scheme cases. This indicated increased costs by influencing the probability of hospital admission for health services and need for monitoring by social services.

*Personality and attitude to help* For both groups, those individuals with a more passive-dependent attitude to help had increased expenditure. Such individuals had a higher probability of admission to long-term care settings, which was more costly.

*Other factors* There was again no change in standard provision, with being female, recently bereaved, and located in the inner city all associated with lower expenditure.

*Initial health status* General health no longer appeared as a predictor of cost to the care scheme group.

*Outcomes* In standard provision, quality of care (Q) again was associated with costs, but this time as a squared term, indicating diminishing returns, or a higher cost of increasing well-being at higher levels. Subjective well-being (M) was not apparently related to cost. However for the care scheme, quality of care did not appear to be associated with cost, although there was a negative effect associated with subjective well-being. This is probably indicative of the effect of improved subjective well-being, in reducing the probability of entry to institutional care, or subsequently requiring less resources. Interestingly, improvement in carer stress was associated with higher costs, and, as in the social cost equation, it appeared that for the care scheme a wider range of outcomes were associated with service provision.

## The cost of improving care for different types of case

In this section an attempt is made to further disentangle the ways in which differences in cost-effectiveness between the care scheme and standard provision could be examined. Here an examination is made of their relative effectiveness in achieving different outcomes for older people. The equations in Tables 8.8, 8.9 and 8.12 to 8.15 have been used to predict and compare the costs of care of achieving different combinations of improvements in the outcomes, subjective well-being and quality of life in the two modes of care. The four key improvement categories of 0%, 20%, 40% and 60% in each outcome have been chosen so as to represent 'no improvement', 'a small improvement', 'a considerable improvement' and 'a substantial improvement' respectively. The typologies presented are based upon an 'average' case within the different modes of care, except that the influence of informal care has been included for costs to the social services department and society as a whole. The influence of other service user characteristics, whether alone or in combination, may be estimated by the extent to which each particular attribute, such as anxiety, was shown to raise or lower costs. The results are shown in Tables 8.16, 8.17 and 8.18.

The average cost of achieving various levels of improvement in subjective well-being and quality of care to the social services department for each group is shown in Table 8.16. The costs for the care scheme group have been broken down according to whether or not the older person was living with their family other than a spouse. It is noteworthy that the care scheme cases living with family cost less than half that for other cases, indicating a degree of interdependence in care which, it was noted earlier in Chapter 7, was not evident in the

**Table 8.16**

*Annual costs of outcomes to the social services department of improvements in well-being, £, at 1981 prices*

| | % improvement in subjective well-being | | | | | | | | | | | |
| --- | --- | --- | --- | --- | --- | --- | --- | --- | --- | --- | --- | --- |
| | 0 | | | 20 | | | 40 | | | 60 | | |
| | % improvement in quality of care | | | | | | | | | | | |
| | 0 | 20 | 40 | 0 | 20 | 40 | 20 | 40 | 60 | 20 | 40 | 60 |
| Care scheme — living with family | 504 | 677 | 907 | 460 | 605 | 807 | 551 | 725 | 955 | 515 | 660 | 863 |
| Care scheme — not living with family | 1435 | 1608 | 1838 | 1392 | 1536 | 1738 | 1482 | 1656 | 1887 | 1446 | 1592 | 1794 |
| Standard provision | 933 | 1362 | 1889 | 827 | 1235 | 1741 | 1108 | 1593 | 2175 | 981 | 1445 | 2006 |

comparison group. In comparing costs by group it can be seen that those for the care scheme cases living with family were always lower than standard provision at all levels of outcome. However, for those cases not living with their family, the care scheme was more expensive, except when considerable or substantial improvements in quality of care were achieved. If marginal costs are considered, that is the cost of achieving an additional increment of quality of care, then at all levels of outcome the care scheme had lower marginal costs than standard provision. In part, these lower marginal costs may be attributed to the different care processes operating in the care scheme and standard provision. In standard provision cases appeared to fall into two groups: first, those who remained at home, received relatively low levels of provision and gained only modest improvements in quality of care; and second, those who entered residential care, received very substantial levels of provision and whose quality of care improved considerably. Conversely, in the care scheme group resources were more evenly distributed between individuals, most of whom remained at home.

Table 8.17 indicates the average cost to society of achieving different levels of improvements in quality of care and subjective well-being for the care scheme and standard provision for an 'average case' both with and without a carer. In general, costs to society were higher for the care scheme cases although the difference reduced with higher levels of the two outcomes. In part this reflected the influence of factors such as housing costs, as people remained in their own homes for longer. As in the previous analyses, this does not take account of the outcomes to carers which were more broadly distributed for the care scheme cases, nor indeed of the wider range of outcomes evident in the scheme. However, when the marginal cost of an increase in quality of care was considered, this was usually lower for the care scheme, except at very high levels.

Finally, Table 8.18 examines the costs of the outcomes for the main agencies, health and social care, for an average case. The costs of the care scheme group

**Table 8.17**
*Annual costs of outcomes to society of improvements in well-being, £, at 1981 prices*

| | % improvement in subjective well-being | | | | | | | | | | | |
| | 0 | | | 20 | | | 40 | | | 60 | | |
| | % improvement in quality of care | | | | | | | | | | | |
| | 0 | 20 | 40 | 0 | 20 | 40 | 20 | 40 | 60 | 20 | 40 | 60 |
| | £ | £ | £ | £ | £ | £ | £ | £ | £ | £ | £ | £ |
| Care scheme — with informal carer | 6265 | 6012 | 5932 | 5983 | 5802 | 5795 | 5474 | 5540 | 5781 | 5029 | 5168 | 5481 |
| Care scheme — without informal carer | 5054 | 4800 | 4720 | 4771 | 4590 | 4583 | 4262 | 4328 | 4569 | 3817 | 3956 | 4269 |
| Standard provision — with informal carer | 4368 | 4630 | 4892 | 4368 | 4630 | 4892 | 4630 | 4892 | 5154 | 4630 | 4892 | 5154 |
| Standard provision — without informal carer | 3550 | 3812 | 4073 | 3550 | 3812 | 4073 | 3812 | 4073 | 4335 | 3812 | 4073 | 4335 |

**Table 8.18**
*Annual cost of outcomes to agencies: social services department and National Health Service combined of improvements in well-being, £, at 1981 prices*

| | % improvement in subjective well-being | | | | | | | | | | | |
| | 0 | | | 20 | | | 40 | | | 60 | | |
| | % improvement in quality of care | | | | | | | | | | | |
| | 0 | 20 | 40 | 0 | 20 | 40 | 20 | 40 | 60 | 20 | 40 | 60 |
| | £ | £ | £ | £ | £ | £ | £ | £ | £ | £ | £ | £ |
| Care scheme | 3796 | 3796 | 3796 | 3594 | 3594 | 3594 | 3356 | 3356 | 3356 | 3081 | 3081 | 3081 |
| Standard provision | 2174 | 2483 | 2849 | 2174 | 2483 | 2849 | 2483 | 2849 | 3271 | 2483 | 2849 | 3271 |

Cost totals are net opportunity costs, discounted at 5 per cent. Days spent in private residential care are treated as though they were extra days in a local authority residential home.

again appear lower at higher levels of outcome. Once again the marginal cost of improving quality of care appeared to be lower for the care scheme group.

Thus, we may infer that for the three major cost accounts, the cost of improving quality of care and subjective well-being favoured the care scheme most at higher levels of outcome. Care managed support proved more costly when the outcomes were comparatively less. However, the marginal cost of improving quality of care appeared consistently lower for the care scheme group. This reflected the finding in Chapter 6 that for standard provision the major gains came from admission to residential care.


**Conclusion**

In broad terms we may identify four concluding observations from this chapter. First, in terms of average costs there was little difference between the care management and comparison groups in terms of costs to social services. In a context where there is a tendency towards higher charging policies for domiciliary care it would seem that there would be further advantage to the care scheme group. In terms of costs to the National Health Service and society as a whole there appeared to be a higher weekly cost to the care scheme group, attributable to the lower personal consumption and housing costs of the comparison group, more of whom were in institutional care. Second, in terms of the determinants of cost, a range of health, dependency and social support characteristics of older people consistently appeared to influence the cost of care. The differential pattern of these between the care scheme and comparison group cases reveals aspects of the different services involved. Third, in terms of the outcomes that were associated with costs, it can be seen that a broader range of outcomes were found for the care scheme group. These were indicative of a greater focus upon the subjective well-being of older people and the needs of carers, compared to the more singular practical needs-focused response for the comparison group. Fourth, in terms of the relative cost effectiveness of the care scheme and comparison groups, the care scheme tended to have lower marginal costs (the cost of producing an additional element of quality of care or well-being) and was generally more cost effective at achieving higher levels of well-being for older people.

# 9 Integrated Provision: Bringing Together Social Care and Primary Health Care

## The origins and background of the scheme

There is clear evidence of marked improvements in the care and support provided to older people as a result of the social care scheme. This suggests the 'added value' associated with intensive care management. However, a constraint to further progress in care at home arose from the complexity of the health care needs of some older people being supported. This led to the establishment of a health and social care pilot project as an extension of the original scheme. For many older people the institutional alternative to enhanced community care was not a residential or nursing home place but at the time was more likely to be a long-stay bed in hospital. From the perspective of the staff operating the social care scheme there were needs which were difficult to meet, in particular dealing with incontinence and immobility and managing episodes of acute illness in severely disabled older people without immediate access to health care expertise. There was a need for additional types of skills and knowledge, which were not possessed by members of the social care team, to supply the training and support required by helpers for the wide range of personal care needs that they encountered. It was considered that these difficulties could be most effectively tackled by closer working with staff who had medical, nursing and paramedical expertise. Fortuitously, this perception by the staff of the social care scheme at the time of its review, when it had been operating for about three years, coincided with a desire on the part of the health authority to examine ways of developing community health services for older people.

A joint bid was made by the social services department and health authority to central government for Inner City Partnership funding not only for the continuation of the social care scheme, but also for a pilot extension in one district of a joint health and social care initiative. This funding provided for additional support of a full-time senior nurse, a part-time registrar in community medicine who had previously worked in geriatric medicine, and 25 per cent of the time of a physiotherapist. In order to permit these staff of different backgrounds to develop a team ethos, working closely together in the care of older people, all members of the team were located within the social care team's office within the social services department. This made possible the informal sharing of knowledge and information to improve assessment and care planning. The health care budget also provided additional resources to be spent in a flexible way, as in the original social care scheme. This meant that the costs of care purchased by the team were shared equally between the social services department and the National Health Service.

In order to permit the new scheme to build on the established social care scheme, it was agreed that the responsibility for team management should lie with the existing team leader of the social care scheme. This meant that it was necessary to be clear about issues of accountability. As in a multidisciplinary approach linking care management with geriatric medicine (Challis et al., 1989, 1995) there were three distinct forms of accountability. Figure 9.1 indicates how accountability was organised in the health and social care scheme.

Accountability for day-to-day work with older people was to the team itself and thus to the team leader. Accountability for the doctor in terms of clinical work was established by rendering him an honorary partner of the group practice whose patients were eligible for entry to the scheme. Administrative accountability for each member of staff was to their respective organisation, for the nurse to the nursing manager, for the doctor to the community medicine sector of the health authority and for the physiotherapist to the senior physiotherapist. The accountability for the policy and development of the scheme was to a newly created joint management body of health and social services of which the research organisation was also a member.

Since the registrar was only a part-time member of the team and due to medical training had to be away for certain periods and the physiotherapist was also part-time, it was decided that the nurse should adopt a care management role within the scheme, comparable with that undertaken by the social workers, but that the inputs of the doctor and physiotherapist would be episodic, principally concerned with the functions of assessment and monitoring. Since the nurse took on the full-time role of care manager the hands-on nursing functions were undertaken by existing nurses working in the community. This reflected both the demands of the care management role itself and the importance of avoiding confusion of responsibility between nurses in different settings for particular nursing tasks noted in another home care scheme (Mowat and Morgan, 1982).

**Figure 9.1**
*Accountability in the health and social care scheme*

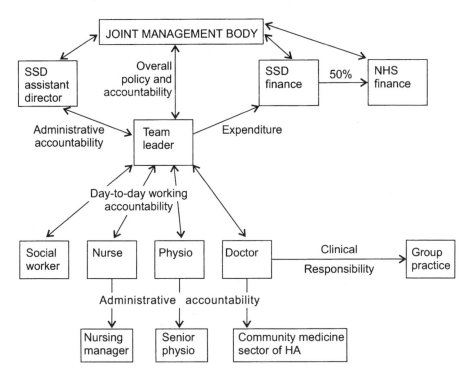

## Care management in the health and social care scheme

This section examines how the core tasks of care management were undertaken in the multidisciplinary model of the health and social care scheme which was organised around a primary care setting. The model is shown in Box 9.1, which indicates that it was a targeted, specialist, intensive and multidisciplinary service.

### Case-finding and screening

The referral sources to the scheme were unrestricted and could come from anyone in the health service, social services or other agencies, as well as from families. The aim was to ensure appropriate referrals by issuing clear guidelines on the target population, beyond specifying that the service was designed to offer a viable alternative to institutional care. These guidelines included which practice the scheme covered, the age of potential clients, the fact that they needed to have multiple health and social care needs, the

---

**Box 9.1**

*Key characteristics of care management in the health and social care scheme*

**Target group** — Older people at risk of admission to residential, nursing home, or long-stay hospital care.

**Intensiveness of care management role** — Intensive care management for a high-need group.

**Location** — Social service department care managers, in specialist SSD team, with outposted community nurse, physiotherapist and doctor as team members.

**Style of care management** — Care managers with responsibility for assessment, counselling, advice and social support, arranging, coordinating, reviewing and developing services and gap-filling.

**Operational features:**
Caseload size: small, 25-30 cases per care manager.
Staff mix: trained social workers, community nurse and community worker as care managers.
Continuity of care: long-term responsibility, undertaking all core tasks from screening to review.

**Influence over providers** — Substantial budget for purchase of external services and items; limited influence to negotiate with in-house providers.

**Management: standards and quality assurance** — Care management team manager carrying reduced caseload; own assessment, review and costs information system; supervision and review using assessment and costs information. SSD team manager responsible for NHS members of team.

**Coherence of arrangements** — Integrated service model for high need group, with nursing and medical expertise integral to team.

---

importance of providing relief to stressed carers, the necessity that home care was a possible means of enhancing quality of life for the older person and that case responsibility for accepted individuals would be taken by the team. One source of case-finding undertaken by the team prior to the commencement of the service was the development of a postal survey similar to work carried out in other areas as a means of uncovering unmet need (Barber et al., 1980; Bowns et al., 1991). Of the 29 cases monitored during the research phase, sixteen cases came via the general practitioner or district nurse and eleven came via the social services department, two of these jointly referred with the health services. Several cases had multiple sources of referral and only four individuals came purely from sources outside the health and social services, such as housing wardens or the survey itself. The characteristics of those people accepted for the health and social care scheme are shown in Table 9.1. It can be seen that they were on the whole more dependent than their counterparts in the social care scheme. In particular all the informal carers appeared to be stressed, and a higher proportion suffered from incontinence and confusional states. A similar proportion, however, experienced difficulty with key activities of daily living.

**Table 9.1**
*Characteristics of the older people supported by the health and social care scheme*[a]

| | |
|---|---|
| Mean age | 80 |
| *Gender* | |
| Male | 20% |
| Female | 80% |
| *Living group* | |
| Alone | 69% |
| Spouse | 17% |
| Family | 14% |
| *Incontinence* | |
| Urine | 48% |
| Faeces | 16% |
| Risk of falling (high) | 53% |
| Presence of confusional state | 48% |
| *Activities of daily living requiring assistance* | |
| Moving indoors on level | 36% |
| Preparing meals | 93% |
| Making hot drinks | 72% |
| Dressing/undressing | 70% |
| Feeding self | 21% |
| Managing medication | 72% |
| Bathing | 96% |
| Shopping | 100% |
| Cleaning | 100% |
| Getting to/using toilet | 54% |
| Getting in/out of bed/chair | 57% |
| Has carer | 73% |
| Carer under stress | 100%[b] |

a Based on 30 cases.
b Of 22 carers.

It would appear therefore that those receiving the service were those for whom it was designed. One important factor in ensuring consistency and appropriateness of referrals for the scheme was the scrutiny of all cases by the team leader prior to their acceptance.

*Assessment*

Using the information available from the referral, the most appropriate individual member of the team to make the first visit was chosen. Thus if the predominant problem was carer stress the most likely person would have been the social worker, but if the major presenting problem appeared to be incontinence it would probably have been the nurse. That first person would then commence the assessment process. In practice this always proved to be the nurse or social worker since they were the members of the team who were to act as care managers responsible for continuing care. Over a period of up to six weeks, depending on the precise needs and difficulties of the individual in question, a person would have been seen by each member of the team: the doctor, nurse, social worker and physiotherapist. The person who had visited first, designated as the care manager, would be responsible for completing the assessment and setting up an initial care plan. It would be their responsibility to work out the most appropriate time for the intervention of other members of the team. Following this period, the team members would meet to discuss each case and to identify whether the problems which had been identified were being tackled suitably, whether there should be a change of care manager and what other interventions or procedures it was necessary to undertake. The team used a common structured assessment format based on that used in the social care scheme, covering activities of daily living, social support, existing levels of care, past history, family stress and relationships, previous medical history and aspects of physical and mental health. This information was collected by the nurse or social workers, and the physiotherapist assessed aspects of mobility in greater detail. The medical assessment was undertaken by the doctor and recorded on a separate document but retained in the same file. When the doctor left the team at the end of his contract, much of the medical assessment role was undertaken by the nurse and focused on physical aspects of health including medical history, medication, blood pressure and foot care. Inevitably, the content of the medical and nursing assessments overlapped to some degree with the social care assessment. Nevertheless, on occasions this more detailed physical assessment identified problems that general practitioners had not identified including sight problems, diabetes, thyroid deficiency and inadequate fluid intake, which were exacerbating other problems.

Within the team setting the 'case conference' was a relatively informal activity. This can be contrasted with a more classical model of multidisciplinary assessment which tends to be hospital or day hospital based where all staff consecutively contribute and a formal case conference is held. In contrast, in the Gateshead model the process was relatively informal and immediate, and decisions could be made and responses sought without waiting for an appointment at a day hospital or a clinic. The very proximity of staff with a different range of knowledge and skills meant that it was possible, in a very informal way, to test out ideas and possible solutions without having to formalise such a process. This was seen by team members as particularly advantageous since it led to a heightened sensitivity to problems beyond the single professional remit. In the case of the social workers it was reflected in an enhanced awareness of the influence of health problems, such as the effects of constipation, chest and ear infections, and for the nurse in a focus beyond nursing inputs and medical condition to factors such as diet, the overall quality of life, the influence of family relationships on care, and the need to vary the pace of work according to the different circumstances of each individual. The care management role and team working influenced all members and the content of their assessments was seen to have broadened to cover a wider range of needs and problems than any one professional had previously covered.

## Care planning

Following the assessment process, which as noted may have taken some time and may have involved setting up of services to tackle immediate problems, the development of a comprehensive care plan took place at a pace according to individual circumstances. As in the social care scheme, the formulation of a care plan reflected a clear hierarchy of need, introduced at a variable pace and reflecting principles of flexibility and choice wherever possible. Often it was necessary to use the monitoring chart to identify the range of care provided at key times of the day and the existence of gaps that required filling. On occasions, existing carers might be under such serious stress that considerable effort was required to persuade them to reduce their input. Consequently, much of the work of building a package of care could at times involve deconstructing the original care system and encouraging relatives to do less. In developing the care plan it was particularly important to recognise how existing patterns of help, although making only a small contribution, could be highly valued and older people, fearful of excessive change and of losing an existing service, could at times be reluctant to receive additional support.

The presence of staff from different disciplines and agencies within the team made it possible to consider and effect more speedily a wider range of responses. For example, the nursing member of the team was able to get immediate access to residential care, day care and other social services facilities, and the social worker could obtain health provided aids and equipment on their own authority. A social activity group organised around meal times was set up in a sheltered housing unit to provide stimulation, companionship and activity to about ten or twelve older people once a week. The team physiotherapist took part in this group and organised a series of simple exercises to music, in order to improve mobility and also monitor progress. It is unlikely that such a simple but flexible use of resources would have occurred in the absence of an integrated team.

As in the social care scheme, the input of specially recruited helpers formed a major part of the care provided. Table 9.2 shows the tasks which helpers undertook in the scheme. The activities were much the same as those undertaken in the social care scheme. However, helpers undertook more personal care tasks, such as managing incontinence, assisting with dressing, and undertook more work in the care of cognitively impaired older people, reflecting the

**Table 9.2**

*Tasks undertaken by helpers in the health and social care scheme*

| Task | Percentage[a] |
|------|------------|
| Companionship and stimulation | 97 |
| Make meals in older person's home | 85 |
| Prepare snack or hot drink | 83 |
| Dressing/undressing | 80 |
| Help with getting up and going to bed | 76 |
| Light housework | 69 |
| Brush or comb hair | 66 |
| Give/check tablets/medication | 64 |
| Clear away stale food | 52 |
| Help with heating system | 51 |
| Help with washing older person | 46 |
| Washing soiled items | 44 |
| Shopping for daily or weekly needs | 41 |
| Change/dispose of incontinence pads/sheets | 40 |
| Take meal from own home to older person | 35 |
| Clean or empty commode, bottle or bedpan | 34 |
| Monitor amount older person has eaten/drunk | 34 |
| Provide reassurance if older person agitated | 33 |
| Reality orientation | 28 |
| Help to use toilet or commode | 18 |

a Based on 4 week period by 22 helpers, percentage of 88 weeks that task was done.

team's acquired experience in this area and the greater proportion of confused people in the scheme.

Helpers were also involved in looking after older people's pets. This latter activity, although apparently trivial, could often be very significant to the maintenance of a person at home and is not normally part of the immediate remit of any agency. Other differences in helpers' activities between the schemes arose from the provision of specialised supervision from team members. Helpers were able to perform a wider range of tasks with training and supervision from the physiotherapist, project nurse or district nurses arranged by the project nurse.

Mrs M. was accepted into the scheme by a social worker in the team. She suffered from multiple sclerosis, was unable to walk or stand and was mobile only in a wheelchair. She had an indwelling catheter and was frequently miserable. She required a substantial amount of practical care and the scheme nurse trained helpers to wash and dress her, change the catheter bag and apply cream to the area. They were also taught to lift her as she was quite a heavy woman. In performing these tasks helpers were acting in place of qualified district nurses, although under supervision, were able to attend at times which suited the elderly woman and also undertake a range of other tasks such as food preparation.

In acting on behalf of other professionals, helpers were performing a role similar to that of multipurpose carers seen in other settings (referred to as home carers, nursing aides and physiotherapy aides) (Challis et al., 1989, 1995). Other tasks which the nurse taught helpers to undertake under supervision included changing dressings, including those for leg ulcers, and condom-drainage. Having the person providing supervision and training as a member of the team appeared to be particularly effective since it meant that they were more readily available for support and guidance.

### Monitoring care

As in the social care scheme, close and regular monitoring of the older person's well-being, the carer's ability to cope and the adequacy and effectiveness of services were crucially important. The usual pattern was one where the care manager, through close contact with the helpers, was able to monitor the situation and this was supplemented by regular visits, often on a weekly basis and very rarely less than monthly. At times, when particular difficulties occurred in the care network, such as conflict between the older person and carers or between different carers, it was necessary for the care manager to become involved directly to resolve these difficulties. At other times, whether dealing with practical or psychological problems, the care manager could work indirectly through helpers and other care-givers.

### Case review: care manager activities and resources deployed

During the period of monitoring the health and social care scheme 33 older people received care from the scheme. Each of these could receive up to three reviews, depending on the period of time they were in the community over one year. There were 78 case reviews in all and the information from reviews one to three has been combined in these analyses.

Table 9.3 indicates the activities undertaken by care managers in the health and social care scheme. The case review format was slightly different from that used in the social care scheme in that activities were categorised by the person or agency with whom the care manager was undertaking them. The activities are broken down into those undertaken with the older person, those undertaken with the informal network, those undertaken with scheme helpers and those undertaken with the formal network.

Almost all reviews noted assessment and re-assessment as an activity performed by the care manager (96 per cent), a higher proportion than in the social care scheme. Three-quarters of the reviews note providing information and advice (74 per cent), which is also higher than the numbers noted in the

**Table 9.3**

*Care managers' activities in the health and social care scheme*

| Activity | Percentage of reviews |
|---|---|
| **With older person** | |
| Support/monitoring | 98 |
| Assess/re-assess | 96 |
| Care planning | 83 |
| Information/advice | 74 |
| Emotional needs | 46 |
| Directing/negotiating older person behaviour | 31 |
| Work with older person in groups/outings | 24 |
| Negotiations with agencies | 24 |
| Escorting | 18 |
| Personal care tasks | 15 |
| **With helpers** | |
| Information exchange | 96 |
| Regular supervision/monitoring helpers | 90 |
| Emotional support/outlet | 76 |
| Temporary/minor changes/relief cover | 74 |
| Supporting/reinforcing helper role with older person | 59 |
| Integrating helper role with informal network | 53 |
| Matching/introduction to older person | 51 |
| Education in skills/tasks/understanding | 47 |
| Integrating helper role with formal network | 47 |
| Helping with day groups | 18 |
| Major change/intervention in helper role/tasks | 17 |
| **Informal network related** | |
| Information exchange | 87 |
| Emotional support | 50 |
| Evaluation of carer need | 45 |
| Evaluation of older person need | 31 |
| Advocacy over older person interests | 28 |
| **Formal network related** | |
| Information exchange | 95 |
| Negotiation over change in service | 32 |

social care scheme. These activities undertaken by the care managers, as well as those of support and monitoring (98 per cent), care planning (83 per cent), counselling, directing and negotiating behaviour and responding to older people's emotional needs can be seen as central tasks of care management (Steinberg and Carter, 1983). The main activities performed by the care manager in relation to the helpers were those of coordinating the helpers' inputs and activities through supervision and monitoring (90 per cent), exchanging information (96 per cent), education and teaching particular skills (47 per cent), providing emotional support (76 per cent), and generally facilitating relationships between helpers, other services and families. These can be seen as key activities in constructing the overall packages of care with particular inputs interwoven from the budget. It is perhaps not surprising that the main activity of the care manager in relation to the older person's informal network was that of providing support to the family. Indeed, providing support to stressed carers of very frail older people was one of the key objectives of the health and social care scheme, as it was in the original social care scheme. Thus, regular contact with the family of the older person or their informal network was noted on some 83 per cent of case review forms. A particularly important task was to ensure that the family understood the level of support and care which was being provided and the reasons underlying particular treatments and forms of help. This exchange of information with the informal network was noted in 87 per cent of reviews. With regard to work with the formal network, the main activities performed by the care manager were associated with exchanging information (95 per cent), which involved ensuring that all the different parties in the care network were aware of and understood the contribution of others so that the support system worked effectively on behalf of the person, and also organising changes in service levels (32 per cent).

Table 9.4 indicates the care managers' contact with different formal agencies. The central importance of health-related problems in this group of particularly frail older people is shown by the degree of contact with a range of different health service providers. Thus, contact with general practitioners occurred in 87 per cent of care reviews, which compares with only two-thirds in the social care scheme. Of course, part of the reason for this could be the fact

**Table 9.4**
*Care managers' contact with formal agencies in the health and social care scheme*

| Formal agency | Percentage of reviews |
|---|---|
| General practitioner | 87 |
| Home help organiser | 70 |
| District nurse | 49 |
| Warden | 32 |
| Hospital inpatients | 27 |
| SSD district office | 27 |
| Meals-on-wheels | 26 |
| Hospital outpatients | 19 |
| Other SSD staff | 16 |
| Other | 15 |

that the health care scheme was located in one specific group practice, which would of itself tend to increase contact with general practitioners.

Contact with the community nursing service was also noted in almost half of the reviews reflecting the fact that for a substantial number of cases, dealing with incontinence and pressure sores required continuing nursing involvement to provide support in the community. Contact with hospitals also proved to be important. The most frequently noted contact within the social services department, as might be expected, proved to be the home care manager to arrange additional home care.

Table 9.5 indicates the main resources deployed in the support of older people in the health and social care scheme. Again the percentage refers to the percentage of reviews in which the particular resource was noted. It can be seen that nearly all cases, throughout the monitoring period, received a paid helper and most cases were in receipt of home help, mentioned in 78 per cent of

**Table 9.5**
*Resources used by the care managers in the health and social care scheme*

| Resource | Percentage of reviews |
|---|---|
| *Domiciliary* | |
| Home help | 78 |
| Aids for mobility | 62 |
| Aids for toileting | 53 |
| Meals-on-wheels | 45 |
| Aids for bathing | 40 |
| *Care scheme* | |
| Paid helper | 96 |
| Transport | 31 |
| Social clubs | 28 |
| Aids for household use | 28 |
| Outings | 24 |
| Aids — other | 15 |
| Other | 47 |
| *NHS* | |
| District nurse | 58 |
| Chiropody | 46 |
| Incontinence aids | 32 |
| General hospital — outpatients | 28 |
| General hospital admission | 19 |
| Bath attendant | 18 |
| Hospital discharge | 18 |
| *Other* | |
| Sheltered housing | 41 |

reviews. Community nursing was noted in 58 per cent of reviews compared with 39 per cent for the social care scheme, again reflecting the frailty of this group. Chiropody was noted in almost half of the reviews (46 per cent) compared with 26 per cent for the social care scheme. Outpatient attendance was also noted frequently, together with the provision of incontinence aids. The provision of various aids for daily living is noteworthy. Aids for mobility (62 per cent), toileting (53 per cent) and bathing (40 per cent) were particularly important. The scheme provided not only paid helpers but also social clubs, outings and transport as a means of resolving particular problems.

Thus, the information presented above confirms that greater health care problems were encountered with this group of older people. It is clear that the activities required of the care managers were once again of a mixed variety requiring direct work with older people and their families and indirect work both in supporting and training helpers in caring for the person and in liaising with agencies and mobilising resources on their behalf. Once again it is clear that the care management role is far more complex than an administrative role and required the care manager to deploy a wide range of skills (Challis, 1994a).

### Responding to need in the health and social care scheme

The case review material provides an overview of the range and frequency of the problems that the care managers in the health and social care team had to tackle. Table 9.6 shows that these older people faced a substantial range of practical problems. In nearly two-thirds of the reviews problems of acute illness had to be tackled, which was almost twice as many as for the social care scheme. This may be expected due to the increased frailty of the older people but it is also indicative of the significance of acute health care problems occurring during the long-term care of a frail older person. It is also notable that a third of the reviews listed problems of a more emotional nature, such as tackling anxiety and depression (33 per cent) which is again almost twice as many as were noted in the social care scheme. Again, almost a third of reviews identified problems with managing medication.

A range of important activities of daily living required attention. These included washing, bathing, dressing, toileting and making meals or snacks. Improving the social environment of older people by increasing social contact, reducing isolation and dealing with feelings of loneliness were also noted in about one-third of reviews. In relation to carers, a priority task involved tackling problems they experienced, as can be seen in the importance of achieving relief (44 per cent of reviews) and trying to tackle difficulties of inappropriate input by carers (21 per cent of reviews). This latter factor often involved the care manager having to work with carers to reduce levels of input, which were excessive and damaging to the carers themselves.

**Table 9.6**
*Older person problems tackled in the health and social care scheme*

| Problem areas | Percentage of reviews |
| --- | --- |
| ***Older person problems*** | |
| Acute illness | 60 |
| Achievement of relief for carer | 44 |
| Mobility — indoors | 36 |
| Making meals | 33 |
| Anxiety and/or depression | 33 |
| Managing medication | 32 |
| Making snacks/drinks | 32 |
| Feelings of loneliness | 30 |
| Bathing | 28 |
| Inadequate social contacts | 27 |
| Toileting | 24 |
| Transferring — bed, chair, commode | 24 |
| Dressing | 23 |
| Mobility — outdoors | 22 |
| Inappropriate input of carer | 21 |
| Mental confusion | 19 |
| Washing | 18 |
| Difficult behaviour | 18 |
| ***Nursing problems*** | |
| Nutrition | 24 |
| Appetite | 17 |
| Incontinence | 17 |

An example of this was an elderly woman whose growing frailty and anxiety at living alone were causing severe stress to her daughter who was her sole carer. The burden of care was intense on the daughter, who also exhibited symptoms of anxiety and depression, along with general exhaustion, all of which led to problems in her marriage. Nevertheless, she felt duty-bound to travel to her mother seven days a week to provide care. She was not willing to accept domiciliary services as an adequate substitute for the care she could provide, but, faced with marriage diffi-culty and negative effects on her own health, she reluctantly concluded she should persuade her mother to enter residential care. Over a period of time, the care manager was able to carefully substitute a package of care by helpers for the daughter's care, on a gradually increasing basis. After three years this reached the point where the daughter was visiting on a purely social basis, with the instrumental tasks of care being under-taken by others.

In the description of the social care scheme in Chapter 5 it was noted how the more flexible approach had enabled staff to help with problems associated with incontinence, immobility, instability, intellectual impairment and informal care. It would seem that in all of these areas of need the health and social care scheme made further progress possible. First, approaches to assessment were improved, giving access to a wider range of knowledge and, on occasions, earlier recognition of problems and access to treatment. Second, in the area of terminal care the enhanced level of support made it possible for individuals to die in their own homes rather than in hospital care. Third, mobility problems and risk of falling were more readily tackled with the input of the scheme physiotherapist teaching exercises and techniques to assist older people in rising after a fall. Fourth, a more effective response to the problems of very high dependency was possible for such people as those who were chair or bedfast, requiring regular toileting routines or with problems in maintaining continence. For such individuals, where multiple health and social care needs were closely intertwined, and particularly where confusion was involved, a higher quality of care could be offered with the team approach. The following case studies illustrate more clearly the ways in which the health and social care scheme brought together a range of skills to support the very frail.

Mr P. was 71 years old and suffered from advanced Parkinson's disease. As a consequence, his mobility, swallowing, ability to feed, continence and speech were affected. He also showed some signs of dementia and suffered periodic 'petit mal' episodes. He was very thin and prone to recurrent urinary tract infections which led to a risk of dehydration. Mr P. was cared for by his wife, who was also in her 70s and had recently undergone major surgery so was unable to cope with him. The nursing service therefore referred him to the health and social care scheme and Mr P. was supported by the scheme for over two years.

Within the multidisciplinary team, a comprehensive assessment was undertaken involving the doctor, nurse and social worker. The doctor arranged for the regional specialist unit to investigate Mr P.'s condition and, particularly, to examine the effects of his medication.

The nurse was concerned with Mr P.'s need for general nursing care, since he required washing, dressing and shaving daily as well as attention to oral hygiene, medication and pressure areas. Mr P. also needed periodic enemas and help with his incontinence. The nurse was able to advise and support the helpers who undertook these caring tasks and to use the budget to supply incontinence aids not otherwise available.

The social worker uncovered a long-standing marital tension between Mr and Mrs P. that clearly stemmed from well before the onset of his illness. Mr P. could be abusive to his wife and, in response, Mrs P. would talk over him or about him and generally neglect his emotional and social needs. Mrs P.'s motivation to carry on caring for her husband at home, despite persistent attempts to gain more support from every and any service, was felt to be largely pecuniary, and hence ambivalent. The situation was therefore inherently unstable and practical care requirements alone were not seen as sufficient.

The couple were offered support every morning to get Mr P. up, washed and dressed, and every evening he was helped to bed. A range of help from different sources was provided to allow Mrs P. to get out. Every week Mr P. went for day care on one day, to a luncheon group run by the scheme on another, he had helpers sitting with him on a third and on a Saturday evening likewise so that Mrs P. could go to bingo. A friend of the family also sat with Mr P. on another day. Despite all this support Mrs P. regularly complained of being left alone to cope with her husband, which involved the care manager in considerable liaison and advocacy work with all the other agencies contacted by Mrs P. Attempts were made to work with Mrs P. over her feelings towards her husband and his dependency needs, ultimately with the goal of acknowledging that she did not want to undertake this role, and could be relieved, but initially this met with only limited success.

After outpatient and day hospital attendance and following some acute admissions, owing to the urinary tract infections, Mr P. was offered an intermittent hospital bed. This was to provide relief for Mrs P. and an opportunity for the hospital to review and stabilise his condition and alter medication if required. With the onset of regular relief in hospital, it became more apparent that Mr P. seemed happier in hospital, was more communicative and physically a little better. He was allowed more freedom and independence than when at home, indicating the effects the difficulty in the marital relationship had on him. Consequently the care manager focused more strongly on Mrs P.'s ambivalent attitude to attempt to reduce the tension at home, relieve her and to permit her husband a better quality of life.

A second example is that of Miss Q.:

Miss Q. was 70 years old and had suffered from infantile paralysis all her life. She was very thin, never having weighed above six stone, and had been very protected by her large family. At the time of referral she only had a sister still living with her, who had herself suffered from a series of strokes. Miss Q. had fallen and fractured her right femur. She had been difficult to re-mobilise and had been distressed, unsettled and disruptive in the hospital, so her sister had brought her home. Despite district nursing and home help input, the sister was having great difficulty coping, and referral to the health and social care scheme was made.

Miss Q. had taken to her bed, refusing to walk or go to the toilet. She would shout for her sister day and night, requesting errands, complaining of pain in her leg and demanding sleeping tablets. The sister was under considerable strain and tired but had been reluctant to accept advice on how to care for Miss Q. She however, accepted advice from the scheme nurse, who became the care manager and had to work closely with the sister and the helpers who, being in the house, tended to become the butt for the sister's complaints and explosions of temper. This required the care manager to provide continued close support.

It was arranged for helpers to call every morning and evening with the aim of getting Miss Q. out of bed, washed and helped to walk to the toilet and through to the front room as a start at rehabilitation. The times of visits were made flexible so that Miss Q. could be encouraged to be up for gradually increasing periods of time and to suit the sister so that she could rest if she had disturbed nights. The physiotherapist, attached to the scheme, was closely involved in devising an activity programme, as Miss Q. would not fully bear weight on her leg. Helpers also called three times a week to simply sit with Miss Q. so that her sister could get out occasionally and also to enable her to attend her own medical appointments.

Since Miss Q. was not always cooperative about getting out of bed, going to the toilet or even eating or drinking properly, a close watch was necessary on both her diet and fluid intake, particularly in view of her weight, and to monitor pressure areas. With persistence and through the role of the care manager in encouraging, training and supporting helpers, trouble shooting, and intervening between both sisters and acting as a buffer between them and the helpers, it proved possible to make gradual improvements in both the standards of physical care and in the social contacts and stimulation for both sisters.

A third example is that of Miss R.:

Miss R., who was 90 years old, lived alone in a terraced house, and suffered from senile dementia, arthritis and post-hepatic neuralgia. She also suffered from recurrent chest and urinary tract infections. Miss R.'s only relative was an elderly sister living out of the area. Miss R. was referred by her general practitioner to the health and social care scheme on discharge from hospital where she had been treated for dehydration and dietary deficiencies, despite receiving a substantial amount of service. This included home help seven days a week, luncheon club once a week and meals-on-wheels twice a week.

Miss R. was a pleasant chatty lady, prone to periods of feeling low particularly when troubled by the post-hepatic neuralgia. Although at times quite disoriented, she managed fairly well in her house and enjoyed 'pottering', looking at old photographs and going through the items in her drawers.

Following assessment, it was clear that after the home help's visit, she was left alone all day and was most unreliable whether she ate or drank. Initially two helpers were introduced through the home help with whom Miss R. was familiar, and attempts were made to encourage her to eat and drink. This involved setting up a simple fluid intake chart, and also negotiating with the home help over the shopping. As Miss R. was unlikely to be specific about what she would like, similar items had been bought each time. Since shopping had been done at weekly intervals, little fresh food was purchased and her diet was rather routine and unappetising.

There were initial difficulties in persuading Miss R. to drink but this was resolved when it was discovered that Miss R. liked to sit at a table 'properly' laid with her china and entertain. At first, the helpers had to drink as many cups of tea as Miss R. to get her to drink properly. It also became clear that she had a sweet tooth and this gave clues as to how to tempt her to regain her appetite, with fresh food and 'tit bits' brought in each day.

Over time, Miss R.'s arthritis deteriorated further, affecting her mobility, so that her house needed to be re-arranged for her to live downstairs. She required help to get in and out of bed, with washing, dressing and toileting. She also became incontinent and at times also needed feeding. Throughout this time, the scheme nurse was able to monitor her diet and fluids, and train the helpers in lifting, checking on pressure areas and in coping with incontinence when this became a regular occurrence. The physiotherapist was able to teach them simple exercises designed to keep remaining functional abilities intact and to slow the process of deterioration.

After a period of stability, Miss R. eventually deteriorated further in both memory and mobility, and was admitted to hospital during one weekend. There she became very distressed so, with her sister's consent, she was brought home with visits increased to six times a day and she was effectively nursed at home until she died.

## Costs and outcomes in the health and social care scheme

### *Location at six and twelve months*

As was noted earlier in Chapter 2, the only outcome data available in the health and social care scheme is that on location at six and twelve months. The matching of those receiving the health and social care scheme with comparison cases was described in Chapter 2. Table 9.7 indicates the location of older people receiving the health and social care scheme after six and twelve months compared with matched comparison group cases. It can be seen that whereas 71 per cent of those receiving this scheme were at home after six months and 64 per cent were at home after twelve months the figures for the matched comparison group were 39 per cent and 21 per cent respectively. Clearly a far higher proportion of those receiving the health and social care scheme were remaining in their own homes. Indeed it is noteworthy that in comparison with the social care scheme the proportion remaining at home is almost identical although in the comparison group the proportion remaining at home after twelve months is even lower (21 per cent to 36 per cent). This would seem to indicate that despite the greater frailty of those people receiving the health and social care scheme, the additional resources enabled the team to keep even the most frail in the community for longer. This difference could be accounted for by a markedly lower institutionalisation rate for those receiving the scheme. Thus whereas only one individual was in a residential care home after six months and only two after twelve months in the health and social care scheme group, the figures were 43 per cent and 50 per cent respectively for the comparison group.

Clearly the effect on prevention of entry to residential care was very marked. It is also noteworthy that of those very vulnerable cases a higher percentage of those receiving the health and social care scheme died at home rather than in one or other institutional care setting. Not only were those people receiving it more likely to remain in their own homes than enter institutional care over one year, but as might be expected over that length of time a much longer period of time was spent living at home. Thus, the average period of time living at home for the health and social care group was 39 weeks over one year compared with 24 weeks in the comparison group.

**Table 9.7**
*Location at six and twelve months in the health and social care scheme*

|  | 6 months | | 12 months | |
|---|---|---|---|---|
|  | HSCS | Comparison | HSCS | Comparison |
| At home | 20 | 11 | 18 | 6 |
| Local authority residential care | - | 12 | 1 | 14 |
| Private residential care | 1 | - | 1 | - |
| Psychiatric hospital | 1 | - | - | 1 |
| Died at home | 6 | 2 | 8 | 3 |
| Died in residential care | - | - | - | 1 |
| Died in hospital care | - | 3 | - | 3 |
| Total number | 28 | 28 | 28 | 28 |

These figures would indicate that the scheme achieved its primary objective of preventing unnecessary institutionalisation of vulnerable older people and permitting them to remain in their own homes where this was their wish.

## The costs of care

Table 9.8 indicates the costs of care in five categories. Once again, costs are shown at a 1981 price base for consistency. The costs of the care management team consisting of the social workers, community nurse, part-time physiotherapist and part-time doctor have been separated from other costs incurred by the social services department and the National Health Service. However the fourth category aggregates the social services department, National Health Service and care management team costs. The fifth category represents the costs to society as a whole.

The care management team costs include the costs of helpers and other items from the budget deployed by the team which, it will be remembered, was met half by health and half met by social services. The remaining social services costs include admissions to residential care, the use of day care, provision of telephones, aids and adaptations and home help and meals-on-wheels. Appropriate allowances have been made for overhead costs. The National Health Service costs other than those of the care management team consist mainly of admissions to different types of hospital: acute, mainly acute, geriatric and psychiatric. The National Health Service costs also include community nursing, outpatient appointments and the provision of aids and appliances. The costs to society as a whole consist of the costs to health and social services, including the care management team, with capital elements of costs discounted at a 5 per cent rate. The cost of housing and personal consumption by the older person, such as fuel, which are included in the costs of institutional care and therefore have to be allowed for in the costs of care at home, were also

**Table 9.8**
*Annual costs for the health and social care scheme (1981 prices)*

|  | £ | | |
|---|---|---|---|
|  | HSCS | Comparison | p value |
| Care management team costs | 1570 | - | - |
| Other SSD costs | | | |
| (revenue net cost) | 606 | 1899 | 0.001 |
| Other NHS costs | | | |
| (assuming 5% capital allowance) | 1162 | 1584 | ns |
| Care management team, | | | |
| SSD and NHS | 3338 | 3483 | ns |
| Social costs | | | |
| (discounted at 5%) | 5159 | 5070 | ns |

included. The financial costs borne by informal carers have not been included in the estimates due to the lack of specific research interview data. However, it was evident from the social care scheme that the financial costs borne by informal carers were very small whilst their major costs were in terms of the burdens and stresses of the caring process. It was clear that the care scheme played an important part in reducing the latter.

It can be seen from Table 9.8 that the annual costs, other than those of the care management team borne by the social services department, were significantly lower for those older people receiving the health and social care scheme. This was due to the much lower rate of admission to residential care. Although costs to the National Health Service were lower for those receiving the scheme this difference was not statistically significant. Since some of the costs to the social services department and National Health Service are taken up by the care management team, and therefore the overall boundaries between agency costs are blurred, it is helpful to consider their joint cost, including that of the care management team. It can be seen that there was no significant difference between the care scheme and standard provision. It is therefore reasonable to conclude that health service costs, joint health and social service costs, and costs to society as a whole were no different for the health and social care scheme compared with conventional patterns of provision. However there are important factors concealed in these aggregates which are worthy of further consideration.

It is clear from earlier discussion and the location of older people at follow-up that there was a marked shift in the pattern of resource utilisation from institutional care to home-based care. For the social services department there was a significantly lower level of expenditure on residential care to the point where the costs of residential care for those receiving the health and social care scheme amounted to 10 per cent of the costs of those receiving the usual pattern of provision. At the same time those receiving the scheme had much higher levels of home help, five times as much as those receiving the usual pattern of care. There was also a significantly greater amount spent on aids for daily living. For the health service, this scheme led to a significantly reduced level of expenditure on mainly acute forms of hospital in-patient care to the point where the cost was only 13 per cent of that of those receiving usual provision. However, health service costs arising from hospital out-patient appointments increased due to the greater number of consultations initiated as a result of the assessment by the care management team. Unsurprisingly, housing costs were higher for the health and social care group as a component of the social costs since they remained in their own homes markedly longer than those receiving the usual pattern of services.

Comparing the cost to society per week of the health and social care scheme of £132 per week with the estimated unit cost of a geriatric bed in 1981/82, including an allowance for capital of £184 per week, then it would seem the scheme was offering a viable alternative use of resources and given the lessons observed from the social care scheme in terms of quality of life, a better use of resources. Furthermore, the joint cost to the social services department and National Health Service of the scheme per week, including the care management team, was about half the cost of a geriatric bed and less than the gross cost of a place in a residential care home. Care manager time constituted 17 per cent of the costs to the social services department and 11 per cent of the joint health and social services costs, a relatively low percentage cost as an investment in better coordinated and planned care of very frail older people.

Thus, as in the social care scheme, it proved possible to offer very vulnerable older people care in their own homes as an alternative to institutional care at no greater cost than the usual services available to them.

### Factors influencing variations in costs

Tables 9.9 and 9.10 show the relationship between costs to the two main agencies, health and social care for health and social care scheme cases and matched comparison group cases respectively.

Although the same broad range of factors appear to influence cost for both groups, namely survival, dependency and social support, in one of these the effect is in the opposite direction. Thus, whereas the co-efficients for social support in the scheme are negative in the comparison group they are positive. Given the much greater probability of remaining at home with the health and social care scheme, this would suggest that for such vulnerable cases in normal circumstances family support is likely to be a predictor of institutional care, families providing the bulk of the care. Conversely, in the health and social care scheme, staff worked so as to make home support complementary to family

**Table 9.9**
*Cost to health and social services combined in the health and social care scheme*

| Variable type | Cost effect | p value |
|---|---|---|
| **Outputs** | | |
| Survival (weeks) | 46.25 | 0.024 |
| **Quasi-inputs** | | |
| Confusional state | 615.64 | 0.097 |
| **Social support** | | |
| Lives with family | -2166.94 | 0.03 |
| Constant | 1143.6 | 0.23 |
| F = 5.04 | | |
| p value <0.01 | | |
| $R^2 = 0.39$ | | |
| Adj. $R^2 = 0.31$ | | |

**Table 9.10**
*Cost to health and social services combined in standard provision*

| Variable type | Cost effect | p value |
|---|---|---|
| *Outputs* | | |
| Survival (weeks) | 145.68 | <0.001 |
| *Quasi-inputs* | | |
| Health and dependency | | |
| Breathing difficulties | 4220.83 | 0.001 |
| *Social support* | | |
| Presence of carer | 2820.61 | 0.014 |
| Lives with spouse | 6630.26 | 0.001 |
| *Other factors* | | |
| Age | 270.70 | 0.005 |
| Constant | -28689.28 | 0.002 |
| F = 7.46 | | |
| p value <0.001 | | |
| $R^2$ = 0.63 | | |
| Adj. $R^2$ = 0.54 | | |

support, thereby reducing the probability of unnecessary admission to homes and reducing the overall care costs as a consequence.

**Conclusion**

The health and social care scheme offers an example of how social care and primary health care could link more closely in the delivery of community care, reflecting the important role of family doctors in the care of individuals with chronic care needs (Taylor, 1991). It offers one example of how to pursue the process of closer integration of primary and community care, which has been a policy goal for some time (NHSE, 1995; Cm 4818-I, 2000). Interestingly, fundholding arrangements did not seem to promote this. The possibilities for linking care management and primary health care might potentially have appeared greater with the advent of fundholding, but paradoxically, it appears that the only community service found more commonly in non-fundholding practices was social work (Audit Commission, 1996).

The health and social care scheme suggests that there are gains associated with linking primary health care and social care. To this extent the findings are similar to those in other studies (Cumella and Le Mesurier, 1997; Ross and Tissier, 1997; Russell-Hodgson, 1997). However, one theme that consistently emerged was the need for specialist health care assessments of many vulnerable older people over and above the expertise available in primary health care teams. Such an observation is not inconsistent with the objectives of Better Services for Vulnerable People (Department of Health, 1997) and with numerous initiatives to more closely link specialist medical assessment to community-based care (Brocklehurst et al., 1978; Peet et al., 1994; Sharma et al., 1994), as has been developed in Australia (Challis et al., 1995, 1998a). Such an approach to integration, a persistent theme in policy documents (Cm 3807, 1997; Cm 4169, 1998; Department of Health, 1998b), can be likened to vertical integration, bringing together service elements at different stages in the production process, as a way of creating effective partnerships between health and social care (Challis et al., 1998a). These and related service development and policy conclusions are discussed further in the next chapter.

# 10 Intensive Care Management and Community Care

The book has examined thus far the initial development and evaluation of the care scheme, namely intensive care management involving health and social care. This started as a predominantly social services initiative designed to meet the needs of that agency. The effectiveness of this approach, the social care model, has been the main focus of the research analysis. In recognition of the importance of multiple needs and the requirement for multiple contributions, particularly to assessment, the pilot health and social care scheme was developed in one part of the area covered by the social care scheme. This was the subject of Chapter 9. It is of considerable interest to consider how the scheme has developed subsequently as it evolved into the mainstream of the work of the social services department.

Services may develop and evolve in response to external pressures, such as funding constraints, or internal factors, such as organisational restructuring and managerial change. One consequence of these may be that the original style or focus of a service may be changed, and the service model will no longer resemble that intended. In respect of innovation, a new service model may lose its core elements as it is forced into the organisational mould of the larger mainstream system. Since the Gateshead scheme was cited as an exemplar of care management in the UK community care reforms (Cm 849, 1989, para. 3.3.3), its own subsequent development may enlighten understanding of the broader implementation of the reforms. The extent to which service models remain consistent has been referred to as 'program fidelity' (Teague et al., 1998). In the context of the development of National Service Frameworks in the UK, designed '...to drive up quality and reduce unacceptable variations in health and social services' (Department of Health, 1999, p.3), specificity and integrity of models of care is of particular importance.

In this chapter an attempt is made to summarise the main lessons from both the schemes described in the earlier chapters and then to analyse the subsequent development of the approach within the social services department, both before and after the implementation in 1993 of the National Health Service and Community Care Act.

## Main findings from the scheme

The care management approach, which originated in Kent (Challis and Davies, 1986), was further developed in Gateshead, providing a basis for testing the portability of the model in an urban setting. A care management team of three social workers, one a senior member of staff, was established with their own budget, directly responsible to an assistant director. A pilot health and social care scheme in primary care, linked to a large group practice, added a community nurse, physiotherapist and junior doctor to the scheme.

### Care management in social care

*The service in practice* During the period of monitoring the scheme, 101 cases were referred and accepted as appropriate. They were a frail group with an average age of 81, who were predominantly female, rather more dependent that those in the original Kent scheme. One third suffered from incontinence and cognitive impairment, a slightly higher proportion from immobility and over one half were at risk of falling. Most required help with key activities of daily living and all needed help with household chores. Over two-thirds had an identifiable informal carer, of whom two-thirds were seen as under stress.

Care managers were responsible for undertaking a comprehensive assessment, necessary for the core aim of creating individual, flexible packages of care which were responsive to changes in need. They used a structured assessment form covering a range of health and social care needs. It was evident that the greater flexibility of response available through a devolved budget encouraged more detailed assessments, less constrained by existing service patterns. Individual care plans were based on the detailed assessment, and took into account the choices expressed by the older person and their carers. New forms of help were developed using the budget under the care managers' control. In common with the original Kent scheme, a group of local 'helpers' who could work flexibly were employed, and paid on a sessional basis, to undertake a wide variety of tasks that often do not fall within the remit of traditional services. The range of tasks undertaken by helpers was very wide, involving such activities as ensuring an adequate diet, providing personal care, helping to maintain continence, giving social support, and assisting people with dementia through reassurance and reality orientation. On occasions, helpers worked to improve mobility following a stroke, under the supervision of a physiotherapist. Care managers regularly monitored the care provided and reviewed their cases using a standard format, covering needs, activities, costs and outcomes (Challis and Chesterman, 1985).

*Outcomes* A matched group of older people receiving the usual range of services from adjacent areas within Gateshead provided a comparison group for the evaluation. Ninety matched pairs of cases were identified for comparison. Both groups of older people and their carers were interviewed upon identification and followed up a year later. The costs of services were monitored over a one-year period for both groups.

Whereas 63 per cent of those who received the scheme remained in their own homes at one year, only 36 per cent of the comparison group did so. Similar numbers of each group were in long-stay hospitals, although there was a very marked difference in the rate of admission to residential homes, one per cent compared with 39 per cent. There was no significant difference in the death rates or length of survival between the two groups. However, over one year those receiving the scheme remained in their own homes significantly longer, on average for 43 weeks, compared with only 33 weeks for those receiving the usual range of services.

Use of a range of quality of life and quality of care indicators over one year demonstrated that on all of the social and emotional need indicators, except the overall morale indicator, there was a significant positive gain for those who received the scheme. They were more likely to have improved in terms of depressed mood, loneliness, satisfaction with life, their level of social activity and perception of their capacity to cope. In terms of quality of care and need for help with daily living, reductions of need were consistently significantly greater for those receiving the scheme than for the comparison group.

Carers' lifestyle problems, such as effects on domestic routine and social activities, and psychological factors, such as carer strain, expressed burden and mental health problems, were significantly reduced compared with those receiving existing services.

An analysis of the average annual costs per case revealed that there was no significant difference between the costs to social services, the National Health Service or society as a whole between the care scheme and standard provision. However, irrespective of whether the older person received the scheme or standard provision, the health service costs were lower in the inner city, due to the lower utilisation of acute hospital beds.

### Care management in primary health care

Additional funds were made available to add to extend the existing team of three social workers, by adding a part-time doctor, a full-time nurse and a part-time physiotherapist with a flexible budget split equally between health and social services. This care management service was designed to focus upon the most frail of the previous target population on the margin of institutional care. It was based around a large group practice, all patients receiving the service being patients of this group of general practitioners.

Since this was a pilot scheme with a relatively small number of cases the only outcome data available is that on location at six and twelve months for a small sample of matched cases (28). After twelve months 62 per cent of those receiving the case management service remained at home compared with only 21 per cent receiving the usual services, a similar result to the earlier findings. There was thus a marked reduction in admissions to institutional care and, furthermore, those people who died were able to do so within their own homes. As in the social care scheme there was no significant difference in costs for the care management approach compared with the existing provision of services to similar cases for the National Health Service, the social services department or society as a whole.

In the next section an examination is made of the organisational framework within which the scheme developed and some of the implications thereof, looking at both the evaluation period described above and also subsequent development after the implementation of the community care reforms in 1993.

## The main phases of the development of the scheme

Four key phases may be identified in the development of the scheme, and issues relevant to the implementation of care management are examined in each. The first was the social care scheme, which ran, in its original form, for some seven years from 1981 to 1988. The second phase, which overlapped, and ran coterminously, with the social care scheme was the pilot primary care joint health and social care initiative, which ran from 1985 to 1989. The third phase involved the extension of the social care scheme to a broader geographical area under local management, which continued from 1988 to 1993. The fourth phase has occurred subsequent to the implementation of the NHS and Community Care Act in 1993, and has involved the development of the scheme as part of the provider side of the social services organisation.

Table 10.1 summarises the four phases and indicates the different ways in which aspects of the care management process were organised at each stage. Each phase is discussed in greater detail below.

### Phase I — social care scheme

The social care scheme was devised as a service with a tightly defined target group of those who were at risk of entry to residential and nursing home care. The care management team was clearly defined as a secondary level service, somewhat analogous to the role of hospital services in health care. That is to say that cases were referred and initially assessed by existing social work teams, who would decide, on the basis of that screening process, whether the care management service was the most appropriate response. Following referral and acceptance, the care management team would assume full case responsibility. For effective case-finding therefore, care managers had to establish their main linkages with existing front-line social work teams. Assessment was undertaken by the care managers and tended inevitably to be single discipline focused, although consultation with general practitioners, district nurses, and hospital consultants would take place where this appeared appropriate. The range of care plans which could be negotiated were at the care managers' discretion and approval for what could be provided was the responsibility of the manager of the care management service, within the team. The helpers, who were paid from the care management budget, were paid on a flexible basis, which varied according to the tasks they undertook and the times at which those tasks needed to be done. Supervision of care managers and the review of their cases was wholly undertaken within the team by the immediate manager, who herself carried a caseload.

## *Phase II — health and social care scheme*

The health and social care scheme was designed not just as an alternative to residential and nursing home care but also was particularly concerned with the more dependent population who could have entered long-stay hospital care. Linkage with a group practice meant that the prime source of case-finding was through general practitioners themselves and nurses based in the practice, although in the early stages the team also attempted questionnaire-based screening of the kind developed in Glasgow (Barber et al., 1980; Bowns et al., 1991). The assessment process was multidisciplinary with an initial assessment undertaken by either a social worker or nurse member of the team with subsequent consultation and involvement of others. This worker would continue to act as care manager. The care plans reflected the greater intensity of personal care needs of these older people and helpers were supervised and taught particular care activities by health members of the team where appropriate (Challis et al., 1995). The helpers were paid by task as in the social care scheme and the budgets were fully flexible within the discretion of the team leader, although the span of budget was broader, covering community health and social care. Training and supervision of helpers was also provided by district nurses where this was appropriate for the tasks they were undertaking. Supervision and review were undertaken within the team and was multidisciplinary wherever this was required. Management of the service was within the team by the team's own manager, who also carried a caseload. Supervision was undertaken on both an individual and group basis, involving input of other care managers.

When the agreement between the health authority and social services to jointly fund the scheme came to an end in 1989 one important remaining

**Table 10.1**
*The main phases of the development of the scheme*

| | Phase I 1981-1988 | Phase II 1985-1989 | Phase III 1988-1993 | Phase IV 1993 - |
|---|---|---|---|---|
| **Goals and objectives** | Alternative to residential and nursing home care | Alternative to residential and nursing home and hospital care | Alternative to residential and nursing home care; gap-filling in domiciliary care | Increasing focus on gap-filling |
| **Case-finding** | Team a secondary point of referral | Through GP practice and team's case-finding strategies | Team allocation meetings; response variable due to team practice | Through assessment social workers; criteria interpreted differently according to experience of assessment social workers of scheme; increase numbers of clients with mental health problems and younger physically disabled |
| **Assessment** | Eligibility and assessment undertaken by team | Multidisciplinary assessment by team members | Undertaken by scheme social workers (care managers) | By assessment social workers or jointly with scheme social worker |
| **Care plans/range of help** | Broad, negotiable by team members | Undertook more personal care and tasks supervised by health care staff than in Phase I | Reduced range of services | Gap-filling, often unsocial hours, rather than comprehensive packages in many cases: therefore more service-focused than client-focused; assessment social worker/scheme social worker negotiate care plan |
| **Case responsibility** | Team care manager | Team care manager | Scheme social worker | As for reviews; problems in DCOs acting as key workers |
| **Budgets** | Flexible at team leader's discretion | Flexible at team leader's discretion; covering community health and social care | Reduced flexibility as scheme in mainstream; e.g. loss of ability to do in-home day care | Budget not clearly known by all scheme social workers; technically a helper budget, although virement possible |

| | | | | |
|---|---|---|---|---|
| *Helpers* | Paid by task not time | Paid by task not time; received nursing supervision and assistance | No budget earmarked for training; trade off between care and training | Payment more time-oriented; soon to be merged with home help service — effects? |
| *Reviews* | Supervision and review undertaken by team | Supervision and review undertaken by team; multi-disciplinary review undertaken where needed | Supervision and review undertaken by scheme social workers | Formal responsibility with assessment social worker: de facto responsibility by scheme social worker where helpers constitute most of package; otherwise unclear; focus in some areas on community reviews, neglect of residential or small resource cases where relatives involved — other areas review where private care involved; cost as trigger for review |
| *Management* | Team's own manager | Team's own manager | Loss of central management leading to different approaches in different areas | Provider service manager |
| *Supervision and support* | By team's own manager; group support of other care managers | By team's own manager; group support of other care managers | Peer group meetings organised, lacked focus in absence of management leadership; individual supervision by different managers | Dependent upon provider service manager; lack of systematic case reviews to assist supervision |

outcome was that district nurses would continue to assist in assessment and train helpers as previously, although this was extended to cover all the areas where the scheme was in operation.

### Phase III — decentralised location of the scheme

By 1988 there was concern to look at ways of expanding the lessons of the scheme across the authority. This occurred at the same time as a move towards more decentralised management of services to older people at the district level. The position of the scheme, centrally managed with a narrow target population and a secondary source of referral, was perhaps slightly anomalous in these arrangements. On the one hand, as a service for older people it could be seen to have a place in the local decentralised management. For some staff it was hard to distinguish between the care management scheme as a whole and some of its specific provider and gap-filling activities and, as a consequence, they classified this work in terms of domiciliary care. Such a perception may often occur around care management schemes, where their broader coordinating roles are less readily and immediately visible (Challis et al., 1995). On the other hand, as a small-scale service relevant to only a small proportion of older people, and therefore small numbers, it could also be seen as more analogous to the mental health service in the authority, which remained centrally managed. Arguments in favour of retaining such an arrangement included peer group support and knowledge in disseminating the care management approach, the style of management and the team approach that had developed, offering a means for further expansion. In the end it was decided that the scheme, as a service to older people, should be decentralised and care managers in districts became members of broader social work teams, with some risk of isolation from their peer group of care managers pursuing similar activities. In developmental terms it meant that there was no key managerial figure to oversee and coordinate expansion across the authority (Davies and Challis, 1986). The lack of a centrally based team meant that the staff could sometimes feel neither part of the social work team nor the domiciliary team in the districts, and could be involved in attending meetings of both groups. Peer group support was absent and staff could sometimes feel very isolated. As one member of staff who had worked in both settings observed, 'When we were a team, if we were having a problem you always had somebody to discuss it with who understood what the problem was'.

There were six staff, one in each of the districts operating this new approach, and a larger number of cases received the service as a consequence, approximately 200 older people at any one time. The goals of the scheme appeared to broaden in these new arrangements, the focus on an alternative to residential and nursing home care was retained, but there was also a growing emphasis upon gap-filling in domiciliary services, with a consequent reduction in emphasis upon managing the whole package. There was also a tendency for the target group to broaden in association with these changes, particularly with varied management approaches and styles in the different districts. Case-finding took place in team allocation meetings, which meant that referrals were not always received on a secondary basis, although of course this was variable according to the allocation practice of different teams. Assessments were undertaken by the care managers, usually on a monodisciplinary basis except where they specifically acted to involve a community nurse, general practitioner or day hospital staff. The size of budgets available to care managers was reduced in the expansion of the service and the range of activities for which budgets could be used tended to contract, with an increasing emphasis on the budgets as being only available to pay helpers. This meant that innovative activities, such as in-home day care, were much more difficult to arrange and activities such as training helpers were also less feasible. However, there were some changes arising from service integration which could be seen as beneficial. Closer working relationships with the home care service and with residential care settings increased the tendency for the mainstream service to consider innovation. Thus, whereas there were losses in some of the intensive and highly client-centred work of the scheme, these had to be balanced against some gains in the range and types of tasks undertaken by the mainstream home care service. The care managers, or community care scheme social workers, retained case responsibility and undertook the supervision and review of the whole care package for which they were accountable. In the absence of a specific manager dedicated to care management, supervision and support tended to have less focus and different styles of supervision were employed by different managers, who had a range of other responsibilities within their team. Supervision was made more difficult, in that information about style of work and proposed care plans and cost information were not regularly collected and reviewed as they had been in the social care scheme. Consequently the information which had provided the focus for supervision was not readily available to the new managers. Despite the attempt to arrange lateral support and supervision through peer group meetings, this was not entirely successful in the absence of clear management leadership focused on the development of care management. It follows, therefore, that different approaches to management, targeting and style of working developed in different areas.

## Phase IV — a provider service

Following the 1993 implementation of the NHS and Community Care Act, the social services department was organised on the basis of a separation between assessment and provision of services. The assessment teams were not deemed in principle to be long-term care management teams, being principally concerned with initial assessment, eligibility and referral with prescription to a service provider. Inevitably, with the budget held at provider level, there could be no guarantee that prescriptions would be met, since providers would be concerned with distribution and allocation of resources. Some aspects of provider integration in geographical areas were retained, with residential and domiciliary services for older people under one manager. The number of districts was reduced, reflecting the spread of managers across assessment and providing functions.

The separation of assessment and provision in the department led to a decision to locate the scheme within a provider unit, albeit one that retained its own budget. The provider service tended to narrow the role of the community care scheme from care manager towards that of key worker for a particular subset of services. Assessments were undertaken either by staff in the assessment team or jointly with community care scheme social workers. The practice would vary according to the length of time that the community care social worker had been established prior to the changes. Where a working pattern was established the community care social worker would usually continue to undertake a substantial part of the assessment. Partialisation of the role of the scheme tended to divert the service from its main objectives of offering an alternative to institutional care towards the narrower one of gap-filling where services were unavailable. This loss of focus and narrowing of role was associated with less clear targeting.

Case-finding took place through assessment team social workers who interpreted criteria differently according to their experience of the scheme, leading to greater variability. One of the changes that was evident was increasing numbers of referrals of older people with mental health problems and younger people with physical disabilities. With different parts of the core tasks of care management being undertaken sometimes by different workers it was more difficult to liaise effectively with community nurses, as had developed from the health and social care scheme. Care plans tended in many ways to be more service focused than user focused, consisting mainly of gap-filling, often in unsocial hours. Diffuse responsibility for individual cases, coupled with the involvement of multiple service providers, could lead to lack of continuity of care, duplication of effort and ineffective use of resources. One example was that of a confused woman who was receiving inputs from both community care helpers and the home help service. The helpers would assist her to get ready in the morning and to dress, waiting while she ate her breakfast. At lunch-time a home help, with little time to spare, would prepare food and leave it in front of her. At tea-time, when the community care helper returned, the food was found to be untouched and spoiled. As a result, the helper had to stay longer than the allotted time to prepare a meal since the woman had not eaten since breakfast. In practical terms it meant that the older person saw members of a team of home helps, members of a team of community care workers, a home help manager, a community care social worker and an assessment social worker. In such cases it would have been better if only one service and one care manager had been involved, to minimise disruption from the multiplicity of different caregivers. However, the structure of the separation of assessment and provision militated against this. In the interests of best practice, it was expected that the assessment social worker would prescribe needs to be met, rather than the mechanism to resolve them, as part of a needs-centred approach. Perversely however, the effect of this was to disengage assessment workers from the detail of care planning, with the kinds of deleterious outcome described above. In short, the strict separation of need identification and problem formulation from the specification of solutions — theoretically a logically stepwise process — did not comfortably fit with the effective separation of roles of assessment and care planning for complex cases, which tended to arise from this particular structure.

Consequently case responsibility was somewhat fuzzy, with formal responsibility lying with the assessment team social worker, although in practice responsibility lay with the community care scheme social worker, particularly in cases where helpers constituted a large part of the total package of care. If the situation changed to any great extent then the older person had to be reassessed by the assessor. The lack of clarity of case responsibility also spread over into responsibility for reviews, where duplication again often took place, particularly as the number of reviews had increased dramatically, arising from an increased workload. This is an area where there has been considerable concern expressed (Department of Health, 1994; Cm 4169, 1998). Often for cases with relatively small resource commitments, or in residential care, relatives were relied upon to monitor well-being. Management and supervision were the responsibility of the provider service manager who, with a wide span of control, could only see the community care scheme care management approach as a small part of their overall concerns. The style of supervision was very much dependent upon the provider manager and the lack of regular case reviews and systematic recording, which had been available previously, could only make this task more difficult, since critical information on the costs of individual packages was not available. After a period it was re-introduced in order to meet this deficit. In plans to re-organise domiciliary care services it was decided to agree to re-introduce the maximum limit for expenditure on domiciliary care to equate to that of the cost of nursing home care. Nonetheless, any case reaching such a guideline ceiling would be considered on its individual merits.

One unforeseen consequence of the narrowing of the care management role and the perception of the scheme in service terms was a growing recognition of the value of the flexibility of response to individual need provided by the helpers. Reflecting the need to respond in a more client-centred fashion, there was a growing realisation of the need to shift much of the style of the home help response towards that offered by the helpers.

Thus, the assessment/provider separation meant that much of the responsibility for creating care packages lay with the provider, as did the process of monitoring the adequacy of the care provided. Hence, an apparently logical separation of assessment and provision in practice had extremely unclear boundaries which led to duplication of effort and problems of responsibility, particularly in the later core tasks of monitoring and review. This experience raises questions as to whether any one particular form of organisational separation is appropriate for all cases, or whether for individuals with more complex needs, continuity of the performance of the core tasks of care management is a critical element of effective home-based care. In short, if intensive care management is to be developed to provide an alternative to nursing and residential care, then it would seem to require a degree of organisational separateness from mainstream social care provision to be fully effective.

However, despite the concerns described earlier about the organisational arrangements for the community care scheme, which militated against effective intensive care management, there is evidence that the service remains concerned with the highly dependent. More recently, in 1997, a comparison was made between older people admitted to residential and nursing home care from the community and a group of older people who were currently supported at home by the community care scheme. As shown in Table 10.2, a higher proportion of those with severe cognitive impairment (Morris et al., 1994) received assistance at home from the care scheme compared with those who entered long-term care from the community (p < 0.05). In addition, more of those cared for at home had high physical dependency (Mahoney and

**Table 10.2**

*Comparison of characteristics of community admissions to long-term care and the community care scheme*

|  | Case type | | | |
|  | Community admissions to long-term care | | Intensive care management service | |
|  | No. | % | No. | % |
| --- | --- | --- | --- | --- |
| **Cognitive status** | | | | |
| Intact/mild (MDS CPS 0-3) | 72 | 80 | 20 | 62 |
| Severe impairment (MDS CPS 4-6) | 18 | 20 | 12 | 38 |
| Total | 90 | 100 | 32 | 100 |
| **Dependency** | | | | |
| High dependence (Barthel 0-8) | 16 | 18 | 19 | 59 |
| Moderate dependence (Barthel 9-11) | 22 | 24 | 7 | 22 |
| Low dependence (Barthel 12+) | 52 | 58 | 6 | 19 |
| Total | 90 | 100 | 32 | 100 |

*Chi-square test:*
Cognitive Impairment: $X^2$ = 3.89 p < 0.05.
Dependency: $X^2$ = 20.24 p < 0.001.

Barthel, 1965) compared with those admitted to long-term care from the community (p < 0.001).

Thus, it is noteworthy that even some sixteen years after the initial scheme, itself having undergone several metamorphoses, that cases supported under the community care scheme were significantly more dependent than cases entering residential and nursing home care in the same authority. This would suggest that the relevance of such intensive support programmes remains valid in the post community care reform era (Challis et al., 1998a, 2001).

### Issues for the development of care management

*Intensive care management and integrated care*

Government policy has increasingly concerned itself with more effective and closer integration of health and social care (Cm 4818-I, 2000) and also the theme of prevention, both generally and specifically in the form of prevention of unnecessary admissions to residential or nursing home care, intermediate care and the maintenance of independence (Cm 4169, 1998; Cm 4818-I, 2000; SSI, 2000). The latter is particularly relevant to the differentiation of care management (Department of Health, 1994; SSI, 1997) and in particular to the development of intensive care management. The study would seem to demonstrate that intensive care management, of the form developed in Gateshead and elsewhere (Challis and Davies, 1986; Challis et al., 1995), is appropriate to the prevention and intermediate care agenda. The evidence from both the social care study and the primary health and social care study was that older people supported by a flexible intensive care management service, which controlled substantial levels of resource, could significantly reduce the probability of admission to residential and nursing home care.

Despite the evidence of the effectiveness of intensive care management as a key component part of the policy initiatives, it is striking to note just how little evidence there is of intensive care management in current services for older people. One recent study examined seven key indicators likely to be associated with intensive care management in older people's services: specialist targeted service for vulnerable older people; specialist teams for older people's services; devolved budgets; care management by health service staff; small caseloads; eligibility criteria specific to community care or older people's services; policy of diversion from residential care (Challis et al., 2001). Only five per cent of local authorities had a specialist targeted service akin to intensive care management and of the seven indicators only 23 per cent of local authorities in England had four or more present. It would seem therefore that, despite the requirement for greater differentiation of care management arrangements (SSI, 1997), in order to develop the prevention and intermediate care agenda, few local authorities in England yet have the arrangements in place to permit this development. It is in this context that the findings of the Gateshead study assume particular relevance. Earlier it was noted that the current services arising from the social care scheme are providing support at home for older people with higher levels of dependency and cognitive impairment that those currently entering residential and nursing homes. Furthermore, there was also evidence that carer support was still a very significant part of this development from the social care scheme.

Given the concern to integrate health and social care more closely at the level of the individual patient or service user, it is interesting to consider where the most effective points of integration may lie for intensive care management. For example, although the health and social care scheme demonstrated gains from linking care management with primary health care, the arrangement was probably not typical of a primary health care linkage, as is discussed below. The physician working with the care management team was dedicated to that activity, had no other patient-related commitments to the practice, and had moved from working in geriatric medicine previously. Similarly, the nurse had all of her time devoted to care management and had no responsibilities for providing hands-on nursing to patients of the practice. Consequently, the medical linkage was markedly different from that which would be the case elsewhere. In many ways the effectiveness of intensive care management may be enhanced by providing linkages with specialist, or secondary care level, medical input, since there is a shared target population of the very frail. Many of these very frail people would have received long-stay hospital care under previous arrangements. Linking care management and secondary health care has been shown in Australia both to provide access to specialist assessment expertise in the community and to more effectively link geriatric medicine with community care (Challis et al., 1995, 1998). In the UK linking care management and secondary health care services has been demonstrated as a means of providing intensive home support to very frail older people (Challis et al., 1995). Thus, in differentiating care management and in pursuit of closer integration between health and social care, it may be most helpful to consider different linkages for different levels of care management. For example, intensive care management may benefit particularly from close links with secondary health care and care management arrangements for less frail individuals may benefit most from linkages with primary health care (Challis, 1998; Challis et al., 1995, 1998).

### Linking social care and primary care

There is a long history of front-line collaboration between social services and primary health care staff. The early work was principally focused on the placement of social care staff in primary health care settings (Goldberg and Neill, 1972; Cooper et al., 1975; Shepherd et al., 1979; Corney and Bowen, 1980; Corney, 1981; Pithouse and Butler, 1994). More recently there have been links established with primary health care, which are concerned specifically with the care of older people. Ross and Tissier (1997) described one such initiative of a care management pilot based in general practice with an additional social work appointment as care manager working in two designated general practitioner practices taking joint responsibility with a district nurse for assessment and care management. As the district nurse continued in a traditional clinical role as well as acting as a care manager it is not surprising that there were difficulties in successfully integrating the nurse into the care management role (Challis et al., 1995). Nonetheless, some gains were cited in terms of improved access for assessment and inter-professional working. Similar gains were observed in other care management linkages with primary care (Cumella and Le Mesurier, 1997; Russell-Hodgson, 1997). Interestingly, a general practice attachment, which did not link care management with practices, as the social worker was separate from the care management system, was less successful than the above, although improved working relationships were again noted (Claridge and Rivers, 1997).

Possibly the nearest example to the Gateshead initiative was the Malmesbury integrated community care team, where social workers, nurses and occupational therapists were all responsible for community care assessments. What was particularly noteworthy was the increased role of community nurses in the assessment process, and also their capacity to obtain both health and social services for their patients. The outcome of the service appeared to be improved access for patients to health and social care, improved professional understanding and speedier assessments (Tucker and Brown, 1997). In their review of the relationship between primary care and social services, Rummery and Glendinning (2000) note a number of relevant factors that facilitate or impede effective collaboration. At the managerial level these include different accountability structures, budgeting cycles, geographical boundaries, ranges of responsibilities and the fact that whereas costs are greater for social services the gains appear to be greater for primary care. For primary care staff differences arise from the independent contractor status of general practitioners and different approaches to the management and communication of information. For social services staff there are the problems of organisational isolation, difficulties in providing cover and administrative support. At the more macro level of joint commissioning, the total purchasing pilots provide an example of primary care being in a position to purchase health and social care for their patients. However, there appears to have been a relatively low interest expressed in the purchasing of community services and little success in purchasing integrated health and social care (Mays et al., 1998; Myles et al., 1998).

The Department of Health inspection of social services' links with primary health care (SSI, 1999) suggested that in respect of older people's services social care and primary health care worked on a parallel, rather than a conjoint basis. This led to lack of multidisciplinary assessment, poor communication and duplication of effort. It also suggested that the most crucial links were between social service personnel and community nurses.

The duty of partnership between health and social care, most recently stated in *The NHS Plan* (Cm 4818-I, 2000), builds upon the new arrangements implemented in *The Health Act 1999*. The Act removed obstacles to joint working by permitting the use of pooled budgets, lead commissioning and integrated providers. *The NHS Plan* also specifies that a key measure of these closer working relationships will be the extent to which they provide older people with improved services. Two arrangements are stressed relevant to the present discussion: first, arrangements at practice or social work level to ensure that older people receive a one-stop service, such as basing care managers in practices, and second, integrated home care teams (para. 7.4). Furthermore, a new level of primary care trusts will provide for closer integration of health and social care. These trusts will be able to commission and deliver primary and community health care, as well as social care for older people and other client groups (para. 7.9-12). These proposals are designed to remove organisational barriers between health and social care so that initiatives, such as the health and social care scheme in Gateshead, may be effected without necessitating the range of organisational complexity so as to facilitate good practice as described in Chapter 9. It is sometimes not easy to realise just how far changes have impacted upon perceptions of the normal or the feasible in the care of older people. For example, in a publication entitled *Developing Primary Care: Opportunities for the 1990s* (Taylor, 1991), there is little mention of the health/social care divide among the key issues in primary care. On the other hand, another study contemporary with this, examining the relationship between community care and general practitioners, noted the need to specify the particular but limited role of general practitioners in the community care assessment process (Leedham and Wistow, 1992). It would seem that this is one area where less progress has been made than in the area of organisational arrangements and funding incentives described earlier.

### Independence, prevention and rehabilitation

Prevention and rehabilitation have been two themes whose importance has risen in the late 1990s. The importance of rehabilitation was first evident in the circular *Better Services for Vulnerable People* (Department of Health, 1997) and independence and prevention were made much more explicit in the White Paper *Modernising Social Services* (Cm 4169, 1998). This, for example, includes residential independence — enabling people to live in their own homes, improving and maintaining levels of functioning and supporting carers. It is interesting to note that the Gateshead study addresses all three of these. Both the social care scheme and the health and social care scheme addressed the prevention of unnecessary admission of older people to residential and nursing care. It was quite clear that levels of admission were significantly lower for those in receipt of the enhanced support provided. Prevention of carer stress was evident in improvements in the quality of life of carers receiving the social care scheme. Furthermore, as noted earlier, the service that developed out of the social care scheme continues to place considerable emphasis on the support of people with carers. Finally, both schemes indicate ways in which prevention through community rehabilitation may be linked with long-term care and support. In the health and social care scheme a physiotherapist, who was part of the care management team, advised at assessment on rehabilitation potential and trained individual scheme helpers in particular activities so as to assist in improvement and maintenance of function of older people. In the social care scheme helpers undertook more low level rehabilitative activity with the cognitively impaired, supervised by the care managers and in more functional activities supervised by district nurses. This link between rehabilitation and long-term care in the community can be identified as a way in which initiatives such as the Community Assessment and Rehabilitation Teams (CARTs) in Cornwall could be linked with care management in the spirit of the new partnership arrangements (MacMahon et al., 1998). This is entirely consistent with the Audit Commission recommendation that screening and assessment arrangements should review people's potential for rehabilitation (Audit Commission, 2000).

## In retrospect

In many ways the Gateshead scheme was well ahead of its time. This was recognised in the White Paper *Caring for People* (Cm 849, 1989) and the validity of the developmental lessons remains. Greater choice and user centredness were made possible by the capacity to create flexible services, through the deployment of a very substantial devolved budget. There will of course always be a tension between flexible services on the one hand and the management of large-scale provision on the other, a tension which will require continuous attention to avoid the potentially high transaction costs of micro-purchasing on the one hand and the risk of bureaucratic inflexibility from block purchasing on the other.

There are two other areas of care management policy and practice highlighted in the Gateshead study. The first is the way in which a separation of purchaser and provider roles may negatively impact upon practice. On the one hand, an over formalistic location of care management in a purchaser role may reduce continuity of care, which is essential to long-term support of very vulnerable people. On the other hand, a provider role narrowly conceived may reduce the span of influence of care management and thereby reduce the capacity to effectively management a total package of care (Challis et al., 1995; Lewis and Glennerster, 1996). The second is the debate as to whether care management can be undertaken by someone also fulfilling another mainstream role, such as district nursing, or whether it is a job in its own right. The

UNIVERSITY OF WINCHESTER
LIBRARY

evidence from the Gateshead study and others (Challis et al., 1995) would suggest that 'part-time' care management is associated with role confusion and less effective performance.

Another theme to which the Gateshead scheme is relevant is that of performance measurement. This was made possible on a small scale through the development of a record system, based upon needs, process, costs and outcomes of care. The data from this made possible effective management of a substantial devolved budget at a time when computer systems to perform such functions were yet in their infancy.

If we may draw one central conclusion from the lessons of the Gateshead study, both during the evaluation phases and its longer-term development, it is of the importance of differentiated approaches to care management. The Gateshead study provides a clear example of intensive care management, the most focused approach to care management for the very vulnerable, and the processes and difficulties of integrating into the mainstream system. It is therefore particularly relevant to the developing agenda of intermediate care. It also provides evidence of ways in which primary care and social care may link through care management and of ways in which such linkage may promote the prevention agenda central to current policies.

# References

Abrams, P., Abrams, S., Humphrey, R. and Snaith, R. (1981) *Action for Care: A Review of Good Neighbour Schemes in England,* Volunteer Centre, Berkhamstead.

Abrams, P. (1984) Reality of Neighbourhood Care: the interaction between statutory, voluntary and informal social care, *Policy and Politics,* 12, 413-429.

Allen, I., Hogg, D. and Peace, S. (1992) *Elderly People: Choice, Participation and Satisfaction,* Policy Studies Institute, London.

Applebaum, R. and Austin, C. (1990) *Long Term Care Case Management: Design and Evaluation,* Springer, New York.

Argyle, N., Jestice, S. and Brook, C. (1985) Psychogeriatric patients: their supporters' problems, *Age and Ageing,* 14, 355-360.

Audit Commission (1986) *Making a Reality of Community Care,* HMSO, London.

Audit Commission (1996) *What the Doctor ordered. A Study of GP Fundholders in England and Wales,* HMSO, London.

Audit Commission (1997) *The Coming of Age: Improving Care Services for Older People,* Audit Commission, London.

Audit Commission (2000) *The Way to Go Home: Rehabilitation and Remedial Services for Older People,* Promoting Independence 4, National Report, Audit Commission, London,

Baldock, J. and Ungerson, C. (1991) What d'ya want if you don' want money?, in M. Mclean and D. Groves (eds) *Women's Issues in Social Policy,* Routledge, London.

Bannerjee, S., Shamash, K., Macdonald, A.J.D. and Mann, A.H. (1996) Randomised controlled trial of effect of intervention by psychogeriatric team on depression in frail elderly people at home, *British Medical Journal,* 313, 1058-61.

Barber, J.H., Wallis, J. and McKeating, E. (1980) A postal screening questionnaire in preventive geriatric care, *Journal of the Royal College of General Practitioners,* 30, 49-51.

Beardshaw, V. and Towell, D. (1990) *Assessment and Case Management: Implications for the Implementation of Caring for People*, King's Fund Institute, London.

Bergmann, K. (1973) Psychogeriatrics, *Medicine*, 9, 643-652.

Bergmann, K. (1979) How to keep the family supportive, *Geriatric Medicine*, August, 53-57.

Berman, S. and Rappaport, M.B. (1984) Social work and Alzheimer's disease: psychosocial management in the absence of medical cure, *Social Work in Health Care*, 10, 53-70.

Billings, A.G. and Moos, R.H. (1981) The role of coping responses and social resources in attenuating the stress of life events, *Journal of Behavioral Medicine*, 4, 139-157.

Booth, R.A. (undated) *Reasons for Admission to Part III Residential Homes*, National Council of Domiciliary Care Services, Norwich.

Bowns, I., Challis, D.J. and Tong, M.S. (1991) Case finding in elderly people: validation of a postal questionnaire, *British Journal of General Practice*, 41, 100-104.

Brocklehurst, J. (1978) The investigation and management of incontinence, in B. Isaacs (ed.) *Recent Advances in Geriatric Medicine*, Churchill Livingston, London.

Brocklehurst, J.C., Carty, M.H., Leeming, J.T. and Robinson, J.M. (1978) Care of the elderly: medical screening of old people accepted for residential care, *The Lancet*, ii, 141-142.

Brown, F.W. and Harris, T. (1978) *Social Origins of Depression*, Tavistock, London.

Brown, J. and McCallum, J. (1991) *Geriatric Assessment and Community Care: A Follow-up Study*, Aged and Community Care Service Development and Evaluation Reports No. 1, Australian Government Publishing Service, Canberra.

Brown, L.J., Potter, J.F. and Foster, B.G. (1990) Caregiver burden should be evaluated during geriatric assessment, *Journal of the American Geriatrics Society*, 38, 455-460.

Bulmer, M. (1986) *Neighbours: The Work of Philip Abrams*, Cambridge University Press, Cambridge.

Caldock, K. (1993) A preliminary study of changes in assessment: examining the relationship between recent policy and practitioners' knowledge, opinions and practice, *Health and Social Care*, 1, 139-146.

Caldock, K. (1994) The new assessment: moving towards holism or new roads to fragmentation?, in D. Challis, B. Davies and K. Traske (eds) *Community Care: New Agendas and Challenges from the UK and Overseas*, Arena, Ashgate, Aldershot.

Campbell, J.C. and Ikegami, N. (1999) (eds) *Long-Term Care for Frail Older People: Reaching for the Ideal System*, Keio University Symposia for Life Science and Medicine, Volume 4, Springer, Tokyo.

Carers (Services and Recognition) Act (1995) HMSO, London.

Challis, D. (1994a) *Implementing Caring for People. Care Management: Factors Influencing its Development in the Implementation of Community Care*, Department of Health, London.

Challis, D. (1994b) Case management: a review of UK developments and issues, in M. Titterton (ed.) *Caring for People in the Community: The New Welfare*, Jessica Kingsley Publishers, London.

Challis, D. (1998) Integrating health and social care: problems, opportunities and possibilities, *Research Policy and Planning*, 16, 2, 7-12.

Challis, D. (1999) Assessment and care management: developments since the community care reforms, in the Royal Commission on Long Term Care, *With Respect to Old Age: Long Term Care – Rights and Responsibilities, Community Care and Informal Care*, Research Volume 3, Part 1, Evaluating the Impact of Caring for People, M. Henwood and G. Wistow (eds) Cm 4192-II/3, The Stationery Office, London.

Challis, D. and Chesterman, J. (1985) A system for monitoring social work activity with the frail elderly, *British Journal of Social Work*, 15, 115-132.

Challis, D. and Chesterman, J. (1986) Devolution to fieldworkers, *Social Services Insight*, June 21, 15-18.

Challis, D., Chesterman, J. and Traske, K. (1993) Case management: costing the experiments, in A. Netten and J. Beecham, (eds) *Costing Community Care: Theory & Practice*, Ashgate, Aldershot.

Challis, D., Chessum, R., Chesterman, J., Luckett, R. and Traske, K. (1990a) Case Management in Social and Health Care: The Gateshead Community Care Scheme, Personal Social Services Research Unit, University of Kent, Canterbury.

Challis, D., Chesterman, J., Traske, K. and Von Abendorff, R. (1990b) Assessment and case management: some cost implications, *Social Work and Social Sciences Review*, 1, 147-162.

Challis, D.J. and Darton, R.A. (1990) Evaluation research and experiment in social gerontology, in S.M. Peace (ed.) *Researching Social Gerontology: Concepts, Methods and Issues*, Sage, London.

Challis, D., Darton, R., Hughes, J., Stewart, K. and Weiner, K. (1998b) *Care Management Study: Report on National Data*, CI(98)15, Department of Health, London.

Challis, D., Darton, R., Hughes, J., Stewart, K. and Weiner, K. (2001) Intensive care-management at home: an alternative to institutional care?, *Age and Ageing*, 30, 5, 409-413.

Challis, D.J., Darton, R.A., Johnson, E.L., Stone, M. and Traske, K.J. (1995) *Care Management and Health Care of Older People*, Arena, Aldershot.

Challis, D., Darton, R., Johnson, L., Stone, M., Traske, K. and Wall, B. (1989) *Supporting Frail Elderly People at Home*, Personal Social Services Research Unit, University of Kent, Canterbury.

Challis, D., Darton, R. and Stewart, K. (eds) (1998a) *Community Care, Secondary Health Care and Care Management*, Ashgate, Aldershot.

Challis, D. and Davies, B. (1980) A new approach to community care for the elderly, *British Journal of Social Work*, 10, 1-18.

Challis, D. and Davies, B. (1985) Long term care for the elderly: the Community Care Scheme, *British Journal of Social Work*, 15, 563-579.

Challis, D.J. and Davies, B.P. (1986) *Care Management in Community Care*, Gower, Aldershot.

Challis, D., Davies, B. and Traske, K. (1994) (eds) *Community Care: New Agendas and Challenges from the UK and Overseas*, Arena, Aldershot.

Challis, D., von Abendorff, R., Brown, P. and Chesterman, J. (1997) Care management and dementia: an evaluation of the Lewisham Intensive Case Management Scheme, in S. Hunter (ed.) *Dementia: Challenges and New Directions*, Research Highlights in Social Work 31, Jessica Kingsley Publishers, London.

Charlesworth, A., Wilkin, D. and Durie, A. (1984) *Carers and Services: A Comparison of Men and Women Caring for Dependent Elderly People*, Equal Opportunities Commission, London.

Claridge, B. and Rivers, P. (1997) *Evaluation of Social Workers Attached to GP Practices: Report to Southern Derbyshire Health Authority*, University of Derby School of Health and Community Studies, Derby.

Cm 849 (1989) *Caring for People: Community Care in the Next Decade and Beyond*, HMSO, London.

Cm 1523 (1992) *The Health of the Nation: A Consultative Document for Health in England*, HMSO, London.

Cm 3807 (1997) *The New NHS: Modern, Dependable*, The Stationery Office, London.

Cm 4169 (1998) *Modernising Social Services. Promoting Independence, Improving Protection, Raising Standards*, The Stationery Office, London.

Cm 4818-I (2000) *The NHS Plan. A Plan for Investment. A Plan for Reform*, The Stationery Office, London.

Collins, A.H. and Pancoast, D.L. (1976) *Natural Helping Networks: A Strategy for Prevention*, National Association of Social Workers, Washington D.C.

Cooper, B., Harwin, B., Depla, C. and Shepherd, M. (1975) Mental health care in the community: an evaluative study, *Psychological Medicine*, 5, 372-381.

Corney, R. (1981) Social work effectiveness in the management of depressed women: a clinical trial, *Psychological Medicine*, 11, 417-424.

Corney, R. and Bowen, B. (1980) Referrals to social workers: a comparative study of a local authority intake scheme with a general practice attachment, *Journal of the Royal College of General Practitioners*, 30, 139-147.

Cumella, A. and Le Mesurier, N. (1997) *Social Work in Practice: An Evaluation of Social Work in GP Practices in South Worcestershire*, Martley Press, Worcester.

Davies, B. (1992) *Care Management, Equity and Efficiency: The International Experience*, Personal Social Services Research Unit, University of Kent, Canterbury.

Davies, B.P. and Challis, D.J. (1981) A production-relations evaluation of the meeting of needs in the community care projects, in E.M. Goldberg and N. Connelly (eds) *Evaluative Research in Social Care*, Heinemann, London.

Davies, B.P. and Challis, D.J. (1986) *Matching Resources to Needs in Community Care: An Evaluated Demonstration of a Long-Term Care Model*, Gower, Aldershot.

Department of Community Services (1986) *Nursing Homes and Hostels Review*, Australian Government Publishing Service, Canberra.

Department of Employment (1982) *Family Expenditure Survey 1981*, HMSO, London.

Department of the Environment (1981) *Housing and Construction Statistics, 1981*, HMSO, London.

Department of the Environment (1984) *Housing and Construction Statistics, 1973-83*, HMSO, London.

Department of Health, (1988) *Home Care for Elderly People 1987/88: Gateshead*, Department of Health, London.

Department of Health (1993) *Monitoring and Development: Assessment Special Study*, Department of Health, London.

Department of Health (1994) *Monitoring and Development: Care Management Special Study*, Department of Health, London.

Department of Health (1997) *Better Services for Vulnerable People*, El(97)62, CI(97)24, Department of Health, London.

Department of Health (1998a) *Care Management Study – Care Management Arrangements*, CI(98)15, Department of Health, London.

Department of Health (1998b) *Partnership in Action, New Opportunities for Joint Working between Health and Social Services, A Discussion Document*, Department of Health, London.

Department of Health (1999) *National Service Framework for Mental Health: Executive Summary*, Department of Health, London.

Department of Health and Social Security (DHSS) (1981) *Care in the Community. A Consultative Document on Moving Resources for Care in England*, DHSS, London.

Dexter, M. and Harbert, W. (1983) *The Home Help Service*, Tavistock, London.

Eggert, G.M., Friedman, B. and Zimmer, J.G. (1990) Models of intensive case management in L. Reif and B. Trager (eds) *Health Care of the Aged: Needs, Policies and Services*, The Haworth Press., Binghamton, NY.

Eggert, G.M., Zimmer, J.G., Hall, W.J. and Friedman, B. (1991) Case management: a randomised controlled study comparing a neighbourhood team and centralised individual model, *Health Services Research*, 26, 471-508.

Evers, A. (1994) Payments for care: a small but significant part of a wider debate, in A. Evers, M. Pijl and C. Ungerson, (eds) *Payments for Care: A Comparative Overview*, Avebury, Aldershot.

Fillenbaum, G.G. (1978) *Validity and Reliability of the Multidimensional Functional Assessment Questionnaire, Multidimensional Functional Assessment: the OARS Methodology*, Center for the Study of Aging and Human Development, Duke University.

Finch, J. (1984) Community care: developing non-sexist alternatives, *Critical Social Policy*, 9, 6-18.

Gateshead Social Services Department (1982) *Budget Statement 1981-82*, Gateshead Social Services Department.

Gibbins, R. (1986) *Oundle Community Care Unit: An Evaluation of an Initiative in the Care of the Elderly Mentally Infirm*, Northamptonshire County Council, Northampton.

Gilhooly, M.L.M. (1986) Senile dementia: factors associated with caregivers' preference for institutional care, *British Journal of Medical Psychology*, 59, 165-171.

Gilleard, C.J. (1984) *Living with Dementia: Community Care of the Elderly Mentally Infirm*, Croom Helm, Beckenham.

Gilleard, C.J., Belford, H., Gilleard, E., Whittick, J. and Gledhill, K. (1984) Emotional distress amongst the supporters of the elderly mentally infirm, *British Journal of Psychiatry*, 145, 172-177.

Gilleard, C.J. (1987) Influence of emotional distress amongst supporters on the outcome of psychogeriatric day care, *British Journal of Psychiatry*, 138, 230-235.

Goldberg, E.M. and Connelly, N. (1982) *The Effectiveness of Social Care for the Elderly*, Heinemann, London.

Goldberg, D. and Huxley, P. (1980) *Mental Illness in the Community: The Pathway to Psychiatric Care*, Tavistock, London.

Goldberg, E.M. and Neill, J. (1972) *Social Work in General Practice*, Allen and Unwin, London.

Gostick, C., Davies, B., Lawson, R. and Salter, C. (1997) *From Vision to Reality: Changing Direction at the Local Level*, Arena, Aldershot.

Gouldner, A. (1960) The norm of reciprocity: a preliminary statement, *American Sociological Review*, 25, 161-178.

Grad, J. and Sainsbury, P. (1965) An evaluation of the effect of caring for the aged at home, *Psychiatric Disorders in the Aged*, WPA Symposium, Manchester.

Grad, J. and Sainsbury, P. (1968) The effects that patients have on their families in a community care and a control psychiatric service — a two year follow-up, *British Journal of Psychiatry*, 114, 265-278.

Graham, H. (1983) Caring: a labour of love, in J. Finch and D. Groves (eds) *A Labour of Love: Women, Work and Caring*, Routledge and Kegan Paul, London.

Green, H. (1988) *General Household Survey 1985: Informal Carers*, HMSO, London.

Greene, J., Smith, R., Gardiner, M. and Timbury, C. (1982) Measuring behavioural disturbance of elderly demented patients in the community and its effects on relatives: a factor analytic study, *Age and Ageing*, 11, 121-126.

Griffiths, R. (1988) *Community Care: Agenda for Action*, HMSO, London.

Hadley, R., Webb, A. and Farrell, C. (1975) *Across the Generations*, Allen and Unwin, London.

Hall, M.R.P (1982) Risk and health care, in C.P. Brearley (ed.) *Risk and Ageing*, Routledge and Kegan Paul, London.

Harris, M. and Bergman, H.C. (1987) Case management with the chronically mentally ill: a clinical perspective, *American Journal of Orthopsychiatry*, 57, 296-302.

Henwood, M. and Wicks, M. (1984) *The Forgotten Army*, Family Policy Studies Centre, London.

Hicks, C. (1988) *Who Cares: Looking after People at Home*, Virago, London.

Hirsch, F. (1977) *Social Limits to Growth*, Routledge and Kegan Paul, London.

Hoenig, J. and Hamilton, M. (1969) *The Desegregation of the Mentally Ill*, Routledge and Kegan Paul, London.

Hoghughi, M. (1980) *Assessing Problem Children*, Burnett Books, André Deutsch, London.

Hoyes, L., Lart, R., Means, R. and Taylor, M. (1994) *Community Care in Transition*, Joseph Rowntree Foundation, York.

Isaacs, B. (1971) Geriatric patients: do their families care?, *British Medical Journal*, 4, 282-285.

Isaacs, B. (1981) Is geriatrics a speciality?, in T. Arie (ed.) *Health Care of the Elderly*, Croom Helm, London.

Isaacs, B. and Neville, Y. (1976) The measurement of need in old people, *Scottish Health Services Studies*, 34, Scottish Home and Health Department, Edinburgh.

Isaacs, B., Livingston, M. and Neville, Y. (1972) *Survival of the Unfittest: A Study of Geriatric Patients in Glasgow*, Routledge and Kegan Paul, London.

Jerrom, B., Mian, I. and Rukanyake, N.G. (1993) Stress on relative caregivers of dementia sufferers, and predictors of the breakdown of community care, *International Journal of Geriatric Psychiatry*, 8, 331-337.

Kane, R.L. (1990) *What is Case Management Anyway?*, Long-term Care Decisions Resource Centre, University of Minnesota, Minneapolis.

Kane, R.L. (1999) Models of long-term care that work, in J.C. Campbell, and N. Ikegami (eds) *Long-Term Care for Frail Older People: Reaching for the Ideal System*, Keio University Symposia for Life Science and Medicine, Volume 4, Springer, Tokyo.

Kanter, J.S. (1989) Clinical case management: definition, principles, components, *Hospital and Community Psychiatry*, 40, 361-368.

Katz, S., Ford, A.B., Moskowitz, R.W., Jackson, B.A. and Jaffe, M.W. (1963) Studies of illness in the aged, *Journal of the American Medical Association*, 185, 914-919.

Keller, R. (1968) *The Urban Neighbourhood*, Random House, New York.

Kendig, H., McVicar, G., Reynolds, A. and O'Brien, A. (1992) *Victorian Linkages Evaluation*, Department of Health, Housing and Community Services, Canberra.

Key, W.H. (1965) Urbanism and neighbouring, *Sociological Quarterly*, 384.

Kivnick, H.O. (1991) *Living with Care, Caring for Life: The Inventory of Life Strengths*, Long Term Care Decisions Resource Center, University of Minnesota, Minneapolis.

Knapp, M.R.J. (1984) *The Economics of Social Care*, Macmillan, London.

Knapp, M.R.J. (1993) Background theory in A. Netten, and J. Beecham (eds) *Costing Community Care: Theory and Practice*, Ashgate, Aldershot.

Kraan, R., Baldock, J., Davies, B., Evers, A., Johansson, L., Knapen, M., Thorslund, M. and Tunissen, C. (1991) *Care for the Elderly: Significant Innovations in Three European Countries*, Campus/Westview, Boulder, Colorado.

Land, H. (1978) Who cares for the family?, *Journal of Social Policy*, 7, 257-287.

Lawton, M.P. (1972) The dimensions of morale, in D.P. Kent, R. Kasterbaum and S. Sherwood (eds) *Research Planning and Action for the Elderly*, Behavioural Publications, New York.

Lawton, M.P. (1975) The Philadelphia Geriatric Centre Morale Scale: a revision, *Journal of Gerontology*, 30, 85-89.

Leat, D. (1983) Explaining volunteering: a sociological perspective, in S. Hatch (ed.) *Volunteers: Patterns, Meanings and Motives*, Volunteer Centre, Berkhamstead.

Leat, D. and Gay, P. (1987) *Paying for Care: A Study of Policy and Practice in Paid Care Schemes*, Policy Studies Institute, London.

Leat, D. and Ungerson, C. (1994) Great Britain, in A. Evers, M. Pijl and C. Ungerson (eds) *Payments for Care: A Comparative Overview*, Avebury, Aldershot.

Leedham, I. and Wistow, G. (1992) *Community Care and General Practitioners*, working paper no. 6, Nuffield Institute for Health Services Studies, University of Leeds, Leeds.

Levin, E., Moriarty, J. and Gorbach, P. (1994) *Better for the Break*, HMSO, London.

Levin, E., Sinclair, I. and Gorbach, P. (1989) *Families, Services and Confusion in Old Age*, Gower, Aldershot.

Lewis, J. (1994) Care management and the social services: reconciling the irreconcilable, *Generations Review*, 4, 1, 2-4.

Lewis, J., Bernstock, P. and Bovell, V. (1995) The community care changes: unresolved tensions in policy and issues of implementation, *Journal of Social Policy*, 24, 1, 73-94.

Lewis, J. with Bernstock, P., Bovell, V. and Wookey, F. (1997) Implementing care management: issues in relation to the new community care, *British Journal of Social Work*, 27, 5-24.

Lewis, J. and Glennerster, H. (1996) *Implementing the New Community Care*, Open University Press, Buckingham.

Lindesay, J. and Murphy, E. (1989) Dementia, depression and subsequent institutionalisation: the effect of home support, *International Journal of Geriatric Psychiatry*, 4, 3-9.

Mace, N.L. and Rabins, P. (1981) *The 36-hour Day*, Johns Hopkins University Press, Baltimore.

McKay, B., North, N. and Murray-Sykes, K. (1983) The effects on carers of hospital admission of the elderly, *Nursing Times*, 30 November, 42-43.

MacMahon, D., McKee, C. and Buckingham, K. (1998) Assessment and rehabilitation teams in the community: the Cornwall experience, in D. Challis, R. Darton and K. Stewart (eds) *Community Care, Secondary Health Care and Care Management*, Ashgate, Aldershot.

Mahoney, F.I. and Barthel, D.W. (1965) Functional evaluation: The Barthel Index, *Maryland State Medical Journal*, 14, 61-65.

Mays, N., Goodwin, N., Killoran, A. and Malbon, G. (1998) *Total Purchasing: A Step Towards Primary Care Groups*, King's Fund, London.

Milne, D., Pitt, I. and Sabin, N. (1993) Evaluation of a carer support scheme for elderly people: the importance of 'coping', *British Journal of Social Work*, 23, 157-168.

Morris, J., Fries, B., Mehr, D., Hawes, C., Phillips, C., Mor, V. and Lipsitz, L. (1994) MDS Cognitive Performance Scale, *Journals of Gerontology*, 49, 4, 174-182.

Morris, R.G., Morris, L.W. and Britton, P.G. (1988) Factors affecting the emotional wellbeing of the caregivers of dementia sufferers: a review, *British Journal of Psychiatry*, 153, 147-156.

Mowat, I.G. and Morgan, R.T.T. (1982) Peterborough hospital at home scheme, *British Medical Journal*, 284, 641-643.

Murray, C., Lopez, A. and Jamison, D. (1993) *Global Burden of Disease in 1990: Summary Results, Sensitivity Analysis and Future Directions*, Harvard School of Public Health, Health Transition Working Paper Series No. 93.06, Harvard University, Cambridge, MA.

Myles, S., Wyke, S., Popay, J., Scott, J., Campbell, A. and Girling, J. (1998) *Total Purchasing and Community and Continuing Care: Lessons for Future Policy Development in the NHS*, King's Fund, London.

National Health Service and Community Care Act 1990 (1990 c. 19) HMSO, London.

National Health Service Executive (NHSE) (1995) *Primary Health Care: The Future. The Debate*, NHSE, Leeds.

Nationwide Building Society (1981) *House Prices Second Quarter 1981*, Nationwide Building Society.

Neill, J., Sinclair, I., Gorbach, P. and Williams, J. (1988) *A Need for Care? Elderly Applicants for Local Authority Homes*, Gower, Aldershot.

Netten, A. and Beecham, J. (eds) (1993) *Costing Community Care: Theory and Practice*, Ashgate, Aldershot.

Netten, A., Dennett, J. and Knight, J. (1999) *Unit Costs of Health and Social Care*, Personal Social Services Research Unit, University of Kent, Canterbury.

Northern Regional Health Authority (1982) *Health Service Costs 1981-82*, Northern Regional Health Authority.

O'Connor, G. (1988) Case management: system and practice, *Social Casework*, 69, 97-106.

Ozanne, E. (1990) Development of Australian health and social policy in relation to the aged and the emergence of home care services, in A. Howe, E. Ozanne and C. Selby-Smith (eds) *Community Care Policy and Practice: New Directions in Australia*, Public Sector Management Institute, Monash University, Melbourne.

Pahl, J. (1994) Like the job — but hate the organisation: social workers and managers in social services, in R. Page and J. Baldock (eds) *Social Policy Review 6*, 190-210, Social Policy Association, London.

Parker, G. (1990) *With Due Care and Attention: A Review of Research on Informal Care*, 2nd edition, Family Policy Studies Centre, London.

Parry-Jones, B. and Caldock, K. (1995) Assessment and practice after reforms: a view from the workshops, a report of the CSPRD Second Annual Conference, *CSPRD Newsletter*, CSPRD, University of Wales, Bangor.

Parton, N. (1994) The nature of social work under conditions of (post) modernity, *Social Work and Social Sciences Review*, 5, 2, 93-113.

Payne, M. (1995) *Social Work and Community Care*, Macmillan, London.

Pearlin, L.I. and Schooler, C. (1978) The structure of coping, *Journal of Health and Social Behaviour*, 19, 2-21

Peet, S. M., Castleden, C.M., Potter, J.F. and Jagger, C. (1994) The outcome of a medical examination for applicants to Leicestershire homes for older people, *Age and Ageing*, 23, 1, 65-68.

Petch, A. (1996) New concepts, old responses: assessment and care management pilot projects in Scotland, in J. Phillips and B. Penhale (eds) *Reviewing Care Management for Older People*, Jessica Kingsley Publishers, London.

Petch, A., Stalker, K., Taylor, C. and Taylor, J. (1994) *Assessment and Care Management Pilot Projects in Scotland: An Overview*. Community Care in Scotland Discussion Papers, University of Stirling.

Phillips, J. (1996) Reviewing the literature on care management, in J. Phillips and B. Penhale (eds) *Reviewing Care Management for Older People*, Jessica Kingsley Publishers, London.

Pithouse, A. and Butler, I. (1994) Social work attachment in a group practice: a case study in success, *Research, Policy and Planning*, 12, 1, 16-20.

Qureshi, H., Challis, D.J. and Davies, B.P. (1983) Motivations and rewards of helpers in the Kent Community Care Project, in S. Hatch (ed.) *Volunteers: Patterns, Meanings and Motives*, Volunteer Centre, Berkhamstead.

Qureshi, H., Challis, D. and Davies, B.P. (1989) *Helpers in Case-Managed Community Care*, Gower, Aldershot.

Qureshi, H., Challis, D.J. and Davies, B.P. (1989) *Why Help: A Study of the Motivations and Rewards of Helpers*, Gower, Aldershot.

Raiff, N.R. and Shore, B.K. (1993) *Advanced Case Management: New Strategies for the Nineties*, Sage Publications, Newbury Park, California.

Ratna, L. and Davies, J. (1984) Family therapy with the elderly mentally ill: some strategies and techniques, *British Journal of Psychiatry*, 145, 311-315.

Romesburg, H.C. (1984) *Cluster Analysis for Researchers*, Lifetime Learning Publications, Belmont, California.

Ross, F. and Tissier, J. (1997) The care management interface with primary care: a case study, *Health and Social Care in the Community*, 5, 3, 153-161.

Rothman, J. and Sager, J.S. (1998) *Case Management: Integrating Individual and Community Practice*, second edition, Allyn and Bacon, Boston, USA.

Rummery, K. and Glendinning, C. (2000) *Primary Care and Social Services: Developing New Partnerships for Older People*, Radcliffe Press, Abingdon.

Russell-Hodgson, C. (1997) *It's All Good Practice: Evaluating Practice Based Care Management in Greenwich*, South East Institute of Public Health, Tunbridge Wells.

Rutter, M., Tizard, J. and Whitmore, K. (1970) *Education, Health and Behaviour*, Longman, London.

Sanford, J. (1975) Tolerance of debility in elderly dependants by supporters at home: its significance for hospital practice, *British Medical Journal*, 3, 471-473.

Schneider, B. (1989) Care planning in the aging network, in University of Minnesota Long-Term Care Decisions Resource Center, *Concepts in Case Management*, School of Public Health, University of Minnesota, Minneapolis.

Seidl, F.W., Applebaum, R., Austin, C.D. and Mahoney, K.J. (1983) *Delivering In-Home Services to the Aged and Disabled: The Wisconsin Experience*, Lexington Books, Lexington, Massachusetts.

Sharma, S.S., Aldous, J. and Robinson, M. (1994) Assessing applicants for Part III accommodation: is a formal clinical assessment worthwhile?, *Public Health*, 108, 2, 91-97.

Shepherd, M., Harwin, B., Depla, C. and Cairns, V. (1979) Social work and the primary care of mental disorder, *Psychological Medicine*, 9, 661-669.

Sheppard, M. (1995) *Care Management and the New Social Work: A Critical Analysis*, Whiting and Birch, London.

Sinclair, I. (ed.) (1988) *Residential Care: The Research Reviewed*, HMSO, London.

Sinclair, I. (1990) Residential care, in I. Sinclair, R. Parker, D. Leat and J. Williams, *The Kaleidoscope of Care: A Review of Research on Welfare Provision for Elderly People*, HMSO, London.

Sinclair, I. and Williams, J. (1990a) Domiciliary services, in I. Sinclair, R. Parker, D. Leat and J. Williams, *The Kaleidoscope of Care: A Review of Research on Welfare Provision for Elderly People*, HMSO, London.

Sinclair, I. and Williams, J. (1990b) Setting-based services, in I. Sinclair, R. Parker, D. Leat and J. Williams, *The Kaleidoscope of Care: A Review of Research on Welfare Provision for Elderly People*, HMSO, London.

Snaith, R.P., Ahmed, S.N., Mehta, S. and Hamilton, M. (1971) Assessment of the severity of primary depressive illness, *Psychological Medicine*, 1, 143-149.

Snow, T. (1981) *Services for Old Age: A Growing Crisis in London*, Age Concern Research Unit, Mitcham.

Social Services Inspectorate (SSI) (1987) *From Home Help to Home Care: An Analysis of Policy Resourcing and Service Management*, SSI, London.

Social Services Inspectorate (SSI) (1997) *Better Management, Better Care*, The Sixth Annual Report of the Chief Inspector Social Services Inspectorate 1996/97, The Stationery Office, London.

Social Services Inspectorate (SSI) (1999) *Of Primary Importance: Inspection of Social Services Departments Links with Primary Health Services – Older People*, CI(99)22, Department of Health, London.

Social Services Inspectorate (SSI) (2000) *Modern Social Services: A Commitment to People*, The 9. Annual Report of the Chief Inspector of Social Services 1999/2000, Department of Health, London.

Social Services Inspectorate and Social Work Services Group (SSI/SWSG) (1991a) *Care Management and Assessment: Managers Guide*, Social Services Inspectorate and Social Work Services Group, HMSO, London.

Social Services Inspectorate and Social Work Services Group (SSI/SWSG) (1991b) *Care Management and Assessment: Practitioners Guide*, Social Services Inspectorate and Social Work Services Group, HMSO, London.

Steinberg, R.M. and Carter, G.W. (1983) *Case Management and the Elderly*, Heath Lexington, Massachusetts.

Stewart, K., Challis, D., Carpenter, I. and Dickinson, E. (1999) Assessment approaches for older people receiving social care: content and coverage, *International Journal of Geriatric Psychiatry*, 14, 147-156.

Sugden, R. and Williams, A. (1978) *The Principles of Practical Cost-Benefit Analysis*, Oxford University Press, Oxford.

Taylor, D. (1991) *Developing Primary Care: Opportunities for the 1990s*, King's Fund Institute and The Nuffield Provincial Hospitals Trust, London.

Teague, G.B., Bond, G.R. and Drake, R.E. (1998) Program fidelity in assertive community treatment: development and use of a measure, *American Journal of Orthopsychiatry*, 68, 216-232.

Thorslund, M. and Parker, M. (1994) Care of the elderly in the changing Swedish welfare state, in D.J. Challis, B.P. Davies and K.J. Traske (eds) *Community Care: New Agendas and Challenges from the UK and Overseas*, Arena, Aldershot.

Titmuss, R. (1970) *The Gift Relationship: From Human Blood to Social Policy*, Allen and Unwin, London.

Tucker, C. and Brown, L. (1997) *Evaluating Different Models for Jointly Commissioning Community Care*, report no. 4, Wiltshire Social Services Department and University of Bath Research and Development Partnership, Bath.

Twigg, J. (1989) Models of carers: how do social care agencies conceptualise their relationship with informal carers?, *Journal of Social Policy*, 18, 1, 53-56.

Ungerson, C. (1993) Payment for caring: mapping a territory, in N. Deakin and R. Page (eds) *The Costs of Welfare*, Avebury, Aldershot.

Ungerson, C. (1994) Morals and politics in payments for care: an introductory note, in A. Evers, M. Pijl and C. Ungerson (eds) *Payments for Care: A Comparative Overview*, Avebury, Aldershot.

Vaughn, C. and Leff, J. (1976) The measurement of expressed emotion in families of psychiatric patients, *British Journal of Social and Clinical Psychology*, 15, 157-165.

Warburton, R. and McCracken, J. (1999) An evidence-based perspective from the Department of Health on the impact of the 1993 reforms on the care of frail, elderly people, in the Royal Commission on Long Term Care, *With Respect to Old Age: Long Term Care – Rights and Responsibilities, Community Care and Informal Care*, Research Volume 3, Part 1, Evaluating the Impact of Caring for People, M. Henwood and G. Wistow (eds) Cm 4192-II/3, The Stationery Office, London.

Wasser, E. (1971) Protective practice in serving the mentally impaired aged, *Social Casework*, 52, 510-522.

Webb, A. and Wistow, G. (1986) *Planning, Need and Scarcity: Essays on the Personal Social Services*, Allen and Unwin, London.

Whittick, J. (1985) The impact of psychogeriatric day care on the supporters of the elderly mentally infirm, in, *Dementia Research, Innovation and Management*, Age Concern Scotland, Edinburgh.

Woodhouse, R. (1992) *Gateshead: A Pictorial History*, Phillimore, Chichester.

Wright, K.G., Cairns, J.A. and Snell, M.C. (1981) *Costing Care*, Community Care/University of Sheffield, London.

Wright, F. (1983) Single carers: employment, housework and caring, in J. Finch and D. Groves (eds) *A Labour of Love: Women, Work and Caring*, Routledge and Kegan Paul, London.

Young, M. and Willmott, P. (1957) *Family and Kinship in East London*, Routledge and Kegan Paul, London.

Zarit, S.H., Todd, P.A. and Zarit, J.M. (1986) Subjective burden of husbands and wives as caregivers: a longitudinal study, *The Gerontologist*, 26, 260-266.

# Name Index

# Subject Index

UNIVERSITY OF WINCHESTER
LIBRARY